# REBOOT:
# JOURNEY OF A TRAUMATIC BRAIN INJURY SURVIVOR

*Getting Through the Tough Times in Recovery and Life*

**A Memoir**

**Evan Higgins**

# Reboot:
# Journey of a Traumatic
# Brain Injury Survivor

## *Getting Through the Tough Times in Recovery and Life*

**Evan Higgins**

Publisher: Evan Higgins
http://on.fb.me/1Swu9kX
https://twitter.com/EvanHiggins

ISBN (Print): 978-0-9963281-0-4

First Edition 2015

# Contents

# Reflections

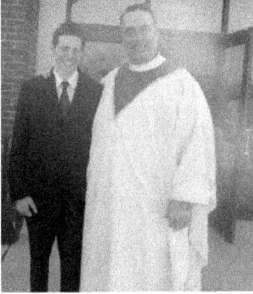

Evan has come a long way since his car accident and he continues to heal and get stronger and healthier. What a great testament of hard work, belief, and love.

Evan was and is surrounded by great family and friends, his sister, his mom and dad, and all his relatives. To go from that day in the hospital when the doctors were losing hope to where he is now moves me and teaches me the power of faith and love, two factors that science and medicine will never be able to explain. Nor will they ever be able to explain that voice I heard in my heart when I visited him in the hospital. I learned many lessons from Evan. It was not just me who brought him the Gospel, he brought it to me in a greater way than I ever could have, because he was the one who had to learn how to walk again, to speak, to remember—to live.

We are blessed when good and beautiful people come into our lives. Evan was all of that and still is to me. I pray that my young friend Evan receives all the happiness in this world and all the grace of our Good Lord. He is an inspiration to me—to us—of goodness, belief, and perseverance. I am grateful to God for giving us the gift of Evan.

*—Your friend,*
*Father John*
*Pastor at Church of the Holy Family*
*Sewell, NJ*

"This is a heartwarming story of tragedy turned into success. Evan Higgins describes his encounter with a life-threatening traumatic brain injury and how he overcame the obstacles associated with his injury and subsequent disability. His determination, motivation, focus, and self-discipline are life lessons we all can and should take to heart."

*—Michael G. Sugarman, MD, FACS*
*Associate Chief, Section of Neurosurgery*
*Christiana Care Health Services*
*Newark, Delaware*

"Evan Higgins has assembled a thoughtful and comprehensive reflection on the life of a wonderful young man who survived devastating traumatic brain injury against odds. In candid form he tells us firsthand of the life before, the recovery and rehabilitation from, and the life after his injury. The very fact that he survived and staged a recovery is remarkable. The fact that he pursued his recovery to the point of being able to author this book is astounding. In my years of practice I have never had such a nearly miraculous recovery as Evan's. Although he still struggles with residual weaknesses, the survival of an intact identity and personality, the love of life and the spiritual realizations his survival have engendered are the real message of his story. I am pleased to have known Evan in the later phases of his recovery and I am impressed with the depth of insight he has condensed into this short but strong reading of his ordeal."

*—Stephen J. Falchek MD*
*Chief, Division of Neurology*
*Nemours/Alfred I. duPont Hospital for Children*
*Thomas Jefferson University*

"I was first informed of Evan Higgins through his mother, Jill, in the fall of 2014. From those first accounts from her of her son's ordeal of what he had been through, I was thoroughly captivated. What completed my astonishment and made me a believer was meeting him firsthand. This is a gentleman and quite the scholar and he is proof that miracles exist. To hear him tell the horrifying details himself kept me mesmerized. I was standing in front of a living testimony of what God can do. Now to have him growing in his faith and spreading his story himself by this book, telling it to audiences and gaining more and more every day the knowledge of the very God who spared his life, it brings me great joy to be a part of this young man's life. You will be inspired after reading this amazing story."

*—Pastor Mickey Robbins*
*Faith Fellowship Ministries Church*
*Malaga, NJ*

# Introduction

After this page, all character names in this book, with the exception of my dad and my neurosurgeon, are fictional to protect everyone's privacy. Everything written is through my interpretations and the information is mostly chronological.

You'll receive many benefits from reading this book. Its purpose is to inspire, motivate, comfort, and give hope to you or someone you know who is facing life's struggles. Just know that you can do it! My hope is that reading this story will help inspire patients, friends of patients, and families of patients to see a brighter, more positive side of them instead of the darker side of a difficult situation they are going through.

This book isn't just for people facing struggles in a hospital. It is an uplifting story for anyone going through a difficult struggle in life, whether from an injury, relationship, educational or work challenge, addiction, or another cause. Only you know what the problem is. Have patience while everything falls into place, allowing you to get through difficult times.

My dad, Robert "Bob" Higgins, said upon reading my book, "If God is first in the equation of your life, all things are possible. No matter what obstacle or trying situation you may encounter or be faced with in your life, large or small, this book will lift your spirit, will increase your faith and will give you the knowledge to realize that miracles can and do still happen."

Dr. Sugarman, my talented neurological surgeon, told me, "Evan, God gave you a second chance in life; He has something very special for you to do. I am going to leave you with the charge to find out what that special thing is and go do it."

# Prologue

On a cold winter day I was driving home after snowboarding with my friend Dan. Dan and I had been friends since the third grade. We gradually grew apart because we were going to different high schools, but we tried to get together on occasion, whether it was to golf, hang out or just listen to music. After snowboarding, I asked Dan for directions on how to get to WAWA, a local convenience store. The roads were decent after the previous day's snowfall. After he told me how to get there, I made a wrong turn and ended up driving on an unfamiliar road. In the blink of an eye, BOOM! My car was T-boned and flew one hundred fifty feet into a cornfield. It was January 28, 2009, a day that entirely changed my life.

# Chapter One
## *Early Life*

*Keep true to the dreams of your youth.*
*—Friedrich Schiller*

As a kid I was always competitive and loved watching and following sports. In the summer, my family and I were looking through videos and found one of me as a kid. It was humorous to see me as a five year old calling my aunt, saying, "Hi. I was reading the paper and the Sharks are leading their division! Did you know that?" Just thinking of how I looked at the stats, watched ESPN and games at such a young age, and continued to do that as I grew up was awesome. My uncle and aunt often brought me to San Jose Sharks hockey games.

I was born in California and lived there until I was six and a half years old, when my family moved to New Jersey. This is where my dad grew up and we had relatives here. I started to primarily follow football, baseball, and basketball, but faded away from hockey.

When I was seven years old, I began to swim competitively at my residential community's private pool. Since we lived just down the street from the pool, I would stay there from early morning until it got dark. I made some great friends and had a blast, every summer casually swimming with friends at practices and then in races every Saturday morning.

When I was a pre-teen I met Ricardo at the summer pool and we became best friends. We were competitive and invested in swimming, so we didn't restrict our swimming to just the summer months but swam competitively in the winter as well. Ricardo was two years younger than me. Once we reached high school we went to rival schools: I went to Schalick High and he went to Woodstown High. We were pretty focused on becoming fast swimmers. Our parents paid for us to join swim teams, practice sessions, and private swimming technique training. Since I was bigger, stronger, and a year older than he was, I always swam faster when we were younger.

During my freshman year in high school I swam with the high school team. After that season I became faster, swimming with older, bigger, and faster swimmers. Being around those swimmers and swimming through more intense practices ultimately made me a faster, more competitive swimmer.

The following summer swim season I started off well, making the "A freestyle relay" and "A medley relay." An "A relay" is the top four swimmers who swim in a relay competing together; when a swimmer finishes his laps, then the next swimmer dives into the pool to continue the race. The freestyle relay is four swimmers racing the stroke freestyle together; the medley relay is a race with a person swimming, in sequence, the backstroke, breaststroke, butterfly, and freestyle.

I remember thinking I was always going to be faster than Ricardo, thanks to high school swimming, my greater confidence and the fact that I was bigger, and stronger. That spring, Ricardo was in gym class and broke his wrist, so he was unable to race at the start of the summer swim season.

The first part of the summer league Ricardo practiced with us, while wearing a special waterproof cast. When we were in the pool, Ricardo tended to swim slower and more casually, pacing himself. I'm sure while his wrist was healing in his cast it didn't give him motivation to swim fast, as he had slight pain with each stroke.

By the middle of July, Ricardo's wrist had healed enough to the point that he was able to compete again. The first swim meet in which he was allowed to compete, he beat me in both freestyle and backstroke races. I was shocked! I wondered, *Why are you faster than me all of a sudden? I was always faster than you in the past and I'm faster than you in practice!* As he got older he became taller and stronger. Most important, he had a really smooth stroke in the pool, allowing him to cruise in front of me. From that summer on, he almost always beat me in a race.

As I became older and faster, I concentrated on having great technique with my strokes. Having good and correct swimming technique allows a swimmer to cruise through the pool with ease. When swimming smoothly, you gain speed. The next year at my high school I was awarded "Most Improved Swimmer." Once I hit my junior year in high school, my times were good and I often took first place in meets.

As a senior, the coach made me team captain. I was given more responsibility to lead my team to victory. I was still an immature high school student, though, so I would joke around with some younger teammates. The coach told each captain to take one swimmer under his wing. Mitch was very tall. He had long arms and legs and had some swimming experience, being a surfer. With his surfing experiences he had very choppy swimming strokes and decided to join the swim team. I saw lots of potential in him and thought, *One day he will become faster than me.*

I took extra time to encourage him, saying he had the perfect body to become great. Since I focused so much on having smooth-form swimming strokes, I wanted to help him with his sloppy surfer-like swimming strokes so he could swim faster. In the beginning, he exerted so much unnecessary energy in the pool that I'd easily cruise past him in practice and races. As time went on, he improved his freestyle stroke, the simplest one for beginners to swim. In January, right before my car accident, he started to catch up with me in the pool.

After the season, while I was in the hospital, I was awarded "Most Valuable Swimmer," even though I missed the last three meets. This award goes to the swimmer who gets the most total points throughout all the meets.

My first job was at the Kountry Kitchen. When I was a freshman in high school, my friend Moe worked at this restaurant as a busboy. He was able to help me get a job as a dishwasher. At first, this was disgusting, wiping off other people's leftover food into the trash and cleaning dishes. After a week, I got used to it, even though this job was redundant and tiring. Constantly, we had to get new carts of dirty dishes, clean them and bring them back to the kitchen. During the five to seven-hour shift, I also had to throw away a heavy load of trash. This job helped me gain a sense of responsibility and good work ethics, working several hours completing the same task over and over. It also taught me the skill of tolerating something you don't enjoy. Having the ability to tolerate a task you don't like can be very helpful for anyone in the workforce. Eventually, I helped a few friends from high school and a few swimming friends get jobs there, as Moe had done for me.

My summer job was lifeguarding at the Elmer Swim Club, the place I called my second home in the summer as a child and teenager. Being a lifeguard was more relaxing and less strenuous on my back, compared to my kitchen job during the school year.

When I was twelve years old, the doctor did an x-ray on my back and diagnosed that I had scoliosis. This was because I had a major growth spurt over a few months, and my posture was awful. I was constantly slouching my spine forward while sitting on chairs and not standing with great posture. After a long day of being on my feet in the restaurant, being a lifeguard was like heaven. Working as a lifeguard helped me gain the skill of patience, having the ability to watch the pool for hours and stay sharp, in case there was a need for a rescue.

I worked all four seasons in high school because my parents told me that I had to buy my first car. With the goal of buying my first car and buying other things that satisfied me, it gave me motivation to work. For anyone, being able to feel that there is a purpose for anything makes the time go by quicker and more desirably.

In high school I made friends easily. I had different types of friends; some were athletic or followed sports, others played music or were artistic. My personality wasn't the nicest and most caring when I was with family and sometimes with close friends. I think it was because I was already outspoken; I wasn't afraid to speak my mind and what I said wasn't always positive.

Years later I spoke to my friend Dan and he told me some interesting opinions and stories on how I was prior to my car accident. Since I've known him for so long and hung out with him often as a kid, I could trust his perspectives on my personality to be accurate. He said, "Sometimes I felt you didn't care what I had to say and you weren't very empathetic. But you were friendly and fun to be around." Also he said, "I knew you for so long, that I understood what your personality was like and didn't take it personally. For instance, if there was something I wanted to tell you that I thought was cool and you didn't, you would say 'I don't care.' It's just something that happens when you are so comfortable with someone." A few other friends took notice of that, but we were still friends. It's common for teenagers to communicate in a rebellious manner and not be mature enough to act like an adult.

In high school I was mostly a B student who was able to slack off and get an acceptable grade. I didn't really need to study that much because my recall skills were sharp enough and I was able to retain information for tests. Not having to exert that much energy to do well in school ought to be considered a luxury that is never taken lightly. If you are still in school or have children in school, be grateful with your current learning ability and always strive to do your best.

# Chapter Two
# Rescue and Rehabilitation

*Miracles only happen if you believe in*
*miracles.*
*—Paul Coelho*

Now we go back to the day that changed my life forever. In the rural farming town where I live, my car was T-boned at an intersection and spun out of control, landing on the front of a house near a cornfield. It just so happened that a local EMT from our town lived in that house. I later heard that he, along with our town's Chief of Police, were on hand to start trying to pull the door down from my crushed car. When other EMTs from our town arrived, I was unresponsive, with just a faint pulse. They used the jaws-of-life to extricate me from the car. When the paramedics arrived, they started giving me medicine to reduce the swelling in my brain. I had to be revived at the scene.

When someone is in such critical condition, they have a limited time to be rescued. If I had stayed trapped in the car, after the rapid shaking of my brain from the impact of the collision that had left me with a severe traumatic brain injury, there would have been no hope for my survival. However, I was lucky. Right before my car accident, two paramedics just happened to be leaving a meeting at the Elmer Hospital, which was only a couple of minutes from where the accident occurred. There also happened to be a volunteer firefighter from a nearby town who came up to that intersection moments after the collision and he called 911. These early divine interventions or miracles were the first gifts that God granted my family and me.

After the EMTs and firefighters extricated me from the car, the paramedics were still performing lifesaving efforts to keep me alive. Since it was foggy, a helicopter was unable to fly me to the closest in-state trauma hospital, Cooper Hospital in Camden, New Jersey. Instead, I was driven to Christiana Hospital in Delaware and placed in the intensive care unit. Before the paramedics left, they told the state trooper they did not expect me to live or even make it as far as the Delaware Memorial Bridge, which was about fifteen minutes away, even though they were going Code 3 with lights and siren. The state trooper notified his commander and a Fatal Investigating Unit was called to the scene.

My parents were notified by the Chief of Police of our town and the state trooper that I was in a car accident and that they needed to get to Christiana Hospital right away. I was seventeen years old. Usually, with a person who is underage, a doctor is supposed to ask for permission from the patient's parents to do surgery. But I was in such critical condition that the neurosurgeon on call, Dr. Sugarman, was going to do the operation even if my parents did not arrive in time to give consent. Fortunately, my parents arrived at Christiana Hospital Trauma Hospital just before the surgery.

Dr. Sugarman met with my parents very briefly in a hospital conference room next to the operating room and said, "As you know, your son was in a car accident. His brain is swelling and his cerebellum is pressing down on his brainstem and I do not expect him to live. He has been given all the medicine to reduce the swelling, but the only thing we can do to save his life is to remove his bone flaps, one on each side of his skull. We do not expect him to live through the operation." As my mom, grief stricken, collapsed onto a chair, my dad asked the doctor, "You have given him all the drugs possible?" The doctor said, "Yes." My dad said, "Go ahead and do the operation."

As Dr. Sugarman was leaving the room he said, "You're doing the right thing; if it were my son, I would be doing exactly the same thing." Before the surgery, Dr. Sugarman didn't expect me to live. I had a Glasgow Coma Scale of 3. This is a neurological scale that aims to give a reliable, objective way of recording the conscious state of a person. For instance, we are all a 15, because we are all healthy functioning people. A 3 is the worst score a patient can have next to a vegetative, brain-dead state, which is zero. If I'd had a 2 on the Glasgow Scale, I'd have been a vegetable. And when a doctor who has done thousands of surgeries in the past isn't optimistic about his patient's living, this doesn't leave the family with much hope for the best.

He told my parents the professional truth. This didn't turn well, especially for my mom; she had a nervous breakdown. My dad was able to hold up better than my mom, but they both cried to the point where there were no more tears, just dry sobs and sounds of grief. My parents and everyone we knew were praying to God for me.

Six hours passed and there were no answers on whether I was going to live or what my life would now become. I found out later that the operation is called a bilateral decompressive craniectomy. In lay terms, Dr. Sugarman had to remove both sides of my skull, each side about the size of your hand, to give the brain room to swell. This was done in order to relieve swelling on the brainstem.

At the end of a ten-hour operation, Dr. Sugarman came out to the OR waiting room and told my dad, "Everything went very well. Your son's vitals were stable throughout the entire operation. He had some bleeds on the brain which we were able to remove, but he also has subdural bleeds that will be reabsorbed by the body. You will be able to see your son in the ICU unit in about 20 minutes." My dad thanked him for everything he'd done.

My parents were able to see me in the ICU room. My dad asked Dr. Sugarman, "With your many years of experience and seeing how Evan's vitals were strong during the operation, if you could give a prognosis on Evan, what do you think it would be?" Without the slightest hesitation, Dr. Sugarman replied, "Cautiously optimistic!" This was the most amazingly positive thing a neurosurgeon could say after a ten-hour operation and after having previously informed my parents that he did not think I would live through the operation.

The next seventy-two hours would tell if I would live or die. During this time, we would see if I could live without life support or if I would end up in a vegetative state. My parents sat vigil by my bedside. Almost at the seventy-two-hour mark, a radiologist called my dad outside my ICU room and told him, "After looking at the CT scan of your son's brain, there is sheering in the front lobe of his brain and some subdural hemorrhaging and we do not expect him to be able to do anything." My father interjected, "Well he's not doing anything now." The radiologist said, "Well that's what we are trying to tell you, Mr. Higgins. We don't expect Evan ever to be moving or out of bed or off any life support tubes."

Now that I had made it past the critical seventy-two hour period, I had to go back into surgery to have my left clavicle pinned together, which was broken during the accident. The doctors also took this opportunity to put a feeding tube into my stomach, which came out the left side of my abdomen. They also gave me a tracheotomy for a breathing tube. My head was wrapped with white gauze around tubes that drained fluid from my head. I had a pin in my shoulder, a feeding tube out of my side, a tracheotomy, and my left ankle was swollen and bruised.

This is how I remained in the ICU for the next two weeks, lying on the bed as a vegetable, with tubes and monitors surrounding me. Eventually I was placed in an ambulance and transported to the local children's hospital and rehabilitation center, A.I. duPont Hospital, in Delaware.

Friends and relatives visited me immediately after my car accident. My friend Gabe, from the Elmer Swim Club, actually had his birthday on the 28th of January, the date of my car accident. He was the first person to visit me in the hospital, once visitors were allowed. Numerous pastors and priests came to visit me and bless me in the ICU. One priest in particular, who came to anoint me and bless me, later told me that, while visiting me in the hospital, he had felt or heard a voice saying that the boy will walk! He was so excited and nervous about hearing the voice tell him this that he could be heard praying for me down the hallway. Later in the book, you will read powerful reflections from that priest describing the experience.

These were the very last words of advice that Dr. Sugarman gave to my parents before I was ready to leave Christiana Hospital: "This is the most difficult time, not for Evan, but for you, the parents. Evan will heal in his own time. My advice to you as parents is this: Don't look behind and don't look too far ahead and that will keep you right here in the present where you need to be, to help Evan with his daily needs." My dad said it was the best advice he could have ever received.

* * * * *

The following is an account of my seven-month rehab, as told to me by my father. When I arrived at A.I. duPont Hospital, I was significantly physically and mentally challenged. I had very little strength, was wheelchair-bound, couldn't speak, and needed assistance with everything I did. As a patient I had three therapies: physical therapy with Nicole, occupational therapy with Zoey, and speech therapy with Samantha. I also attended school and group therapy.

When I first started physical therapy, my friend Ricardo would later say to me, "You were out of it." I wore a protective helmet on my head, which looked like a football helmet from the 1920s, which covered my entire head, since there was no skull bone. I had a neck collar with a special hole in the front part of my neck so I could breathe through the tracheotomy tube. I could not communicate or do anything at all. My brain was trying to heal.

My first day at A.I. duPont Hospital was a long and emotional one for my mom and dad. I was assigned Nurse Susan, who was there to check me into the hospital and who would be my nurse until the time I left A.I. duPont Hospital. Another nurse was also assigned to me, but she was later reassigned, so Lori, the shift supervisor nurse, took her place as my other primary care nurse with Nurse Susan. What a blessing, both nurses took such great care of me and were constantly looking out for me and helping me progress. It was the hospital policy to have one primary nurse who cares for you; that way, there is a continuity of care from someone who knows you and your condition. There was a whirlwind of doctors, one after another, coming into my room doing evaluations and scheduling me for tests.

At one point, a mobile x-ray unit came in and started to turn me to put an x-ray plate under my upper back and neck. My father jumped up and stopped them, saying, "He has to have his protective helmet on before you put that under his neck or roll him!" The technicians hadn't known that I did not have any skull bone, because my head was still wrapped with gauze. My dad was constantly looking out for my welfare.

Because my hands were going all over the place, my dad wanted my hands to be tied to the side of the bed, just like the nurses had done over at Christiana Hospital, to protect me from hitting my head. At A.I. duPont Hospital they reluctantly followed my dad's request. That same first day I was moved to an isolation room, as was standard hospital policy, in case someone had a disease or another contagious condition. Every day my mom and dad drove down from New Jersey to Delaware to be with me. I was finally cleared by the medical staff and taken out of the isolation room and put in a regular room about two weeks later.

The head neurosurgeon at A.I. duPont Hospital was going to perform a spinal tap to find out if the spinal fluid was clear or if it had blood in it. This would tell the treating doctors if my brain was still bleeding or if it was starting to heal. The spinal fluid was a rusty, more yellowish color, which meant that my brain had stopped bleeding and was starting to heal. As a result of the doctors' findings, the doctors felt that they could remove the drainage tubes from my head.

Because this operation was going to be done very early in the morning, my dad decided to stay overnight to be with me as I went to the operating room. My dad works for the state as an operating engineer in a powerhouse, and for the nine years up until my accident he had never called out sick. He was able to use all his accumulated sick time to stay with me in the hospital and help me, twenty-four/seven. From that day forward, my dad lived with me at the hospital and slept on a foldout lounge chair next to my bed.

They explained to my parents that I would start inpatient intensive rehabilitation once I was cleared from the isolation room. Indeed, I started rehab the day after I was taken out of isolation. My brain was trying to heal and find new pathways and connections. My brain did not know how to regulate temperature or any of the other basic functions of life, so one week I was freezing cold, the next week I was sweating profusely. I was fed my meals through a feeding tube by a machine, and I had a ventilation machine to help me breathe. Whenever I was transported to the therapy room, they hooked up a portable ventilator. After a few weeks I was taken off the ventilating machine and used my trach tube to breathe.

My dad said that the physical and occupational therapists worked together during that first day in therapy. They each lifted an arm to start stretching and loosening me up. My dad said that from the expression on my face it looked very painful. The therapist kept asking me if it hurt. They continued to stretch my arms out until I finally said out of pain or anger, "Yes!" That's what they wanted me to do. They wanted to see if I would respond appropriately to painful stimuli, and I did. Then they asked, "Do you want us to stop stretching your arms?" They did not stop until I said yes, and I did. I know it doesn't sound like much for the first session, but it was a long process to get me out of bed, hook up the portable ventilator and get me set up on the therapy platform.

I went to the speech therapist right after my physical therapy. She gave my dad a binder containing my name, age, and birthdate; the name of the hospital I was at; what high school I went to; my home address—all the pertinent information my dad would have to go over with me at night after my daytime speech therapy session.

After speech therapy I went to school. They had a licensed school teacher there who started me off with beginning math and reading lessons. After school I had a break for lunch, which was a measured portion of liquid food fed to me by a machine. I also went to group therapy and a one-on-one session with a psychologist.

By the time all my therapy and classroom and group sessions were done, it was just about a full eight-hour day. This was my routine for five months of rehabilitation. The only thing that changed during that time was the order in which I had the sessions. For the most part, my schedule was breakfast, occupational therapy, speech therapy, classroom studies, group therapy, one-on-one psychologist therapy, lunch, and physical therapy.

# Chapter Three
## *Sudden Improvement*

*When your skull bones were put back into*
*place it was like rebooting a computer.*
*—My dad, Robert Higgins*

It took almost eight weeks for the swelling of my brain to go down. Dr. Sugarman felt I was ready to go back to Christiana Hospital to have my medically frozen skull bones (medically known as bone flaps) reinserted into my head. I was temporarily discharged from A.I. duPont Hospital for the surgery and admitted into Christiana Hospital for this purpose. The operation was basically the same as the day of my accident, except this time I was not in a critical life-or-death situation. After my scalp was folded back then my skull bones, which had been prepared and tested prior to my operation, were then placed back into my head and secured with titanium bolts. I was in Christiana Hospital for about five days, all together, to have this surgery performed, including being in ICU for three days for observation afterwards. I also had drainage tubes in the back of my head until the drainage had stopped; then Dr. Sugarman removed them. At this point I was moved down to a regular hospital room for two more days before being transported back to A.I. duPont

Hospital. All therapy was put on hold for two weeks until my sutures were removed, even though I had been readmitted to A.I. duPont Hospital Rehabilitation Department.

After I arrived back at A.I duPont Hospital, one of the doctors from the neurology department came by, making his rounds on a routine checkup. He saw the newspaper clippings and swimming pictures on the wall of my room and asked my dad, "Your son is a swimmer?" My dad said yes, and proceeded to tell the doctor that I was a competitive swimmer, captain of my high school swim team, and that I normally practiced swimming all year round. He told my dad that an athlete can get emotionally depressed if he is not training and mentally has to get back to his sport to do better after an injury. He said, "As soon as he has his sutures out, I want him in the pool downstairs to do aquatic therapy."

It was nice that I was getting back in the pool, a passion that I'd had before the car accident. I started my aquatic therapy 14 days later by standing in the water, having two physical therapists with me. This was very helpful. Since being in the water is a state of weightlessness, it was the first time I had been able to stand by myself, holding onto the side rail in the pool. This therapy started with standing in the water and using a life jacket to let me float on my back and move and kick with my legs. Later, the therapist let me try swimming laps with a life jacket on.

After a while, I started to get the hang of it and was able to swim like I used to. Of course, being competitive, I wanted to know how fast I was going. Eventually, as I started healing more, I was able to have my dad time me swimming one lap in a twenty-seven-yard pool. With a life jacket and all the safety floats on my arms, I swam in eighteen seconds. I was ecstatic!

While in my therapies, I talked about how I used to be a good swimmer. Adam, one of the therapy aides, came to watch me swim laps. He was amazed at how well I was doing in the pool. My aquatic therapy came to an end when my therapist left on maternity leave. However, the timing worked out for me, because I was able to go home on the weekends and swim at the private swim club where we were members.

My car accident had been in a rural farming area in Upper Pittsgrove, New Jersey. As usual, police officers—in this case a state trooper—had to take notes of what happened, since the accident had occurred on a state highway. As already mentioned, the paramedics did not think that I would make it to the Delaware Memorial Bridge. The state trooper notified his lieutenant, commander of the Woodstown State Police Barracks, and the commander sent out a Fatal Investigative Unit to document the scene.

Oddly enough, in a simple twist of fate, one week later at almost the same time of day, the commander's nine-year-old daughter was in a sledding accident. This accident damaged her brain as well. We both were patients at A.I. duPont Hospital. After the officer realized it was me in the near-fatal car accident and that he also knew my Uncle Sam, a retired captain in the state police, both of our families became friends.

During my stay at A.I. duPont Hospital, my dad was constantly with me. He ended up sleeping in my room when I was going through rehabilitation. He did this because a few years prior to this his dad had suffered a massive stroke. My dad and his sister took charge of helping their dad. My aunt lived in Florida and could be with my grandfather, but my dad took care of the medical insurance and visited his father for one week out of every month to see him and help him.

Unfortunately, he saw the negative aspects of hospitals, regarding insurance and how patients are sometimes treated or neglected, primarily because the hospitals and nursing homes are understaffed. He saw that his dad wasn't cleaned or changed during the night and as a result contracted infections from the improper care. My dad saw that his father was improving and probably could have regained his speech and walking abilities. Instead, from all the infections he had to fight off, my grandfather eventually passed away. My dad and aunt wanted to stay with him all night and take care of their father, but they were not allowed to be with him because he was an adult.

After having this experience with his father, my dad decided that in order for me to have the best possible outcome, he would stay with me around the clock to care for me. He said if he could keep the trach, feeding tube, suture sites clean and free from any infections, also have me cleaned and changed so that there was no skin breakdown from waste products, then my body wouldn't have to fight off any infections. He also cleaned out my mouth from the thrush buildup that occurred from not eating by mouth. He regularly moved and exercised every joint in my body to keep me limber. He thought maybe it would trigger my brain to reconnect the circuit for my limbs to move. Now all my body and mind had to do was heal. Since I was a minor, he had more control, because parents were allowed to stay in the room.

Besides Nurse Susan, who was assigned to me, other nurses always wanted to sign up on the list to take care of me when I was a patient. Perhaps this was because my dad, a local volunteer firefighter and EMT, did a lot of the work, after he was taught by Nurse Susan. For instance, cleaning my feeding tube and setting up the machine and making sure that I was always changed and cleaned with the nurse's assistance, no matter what time of night it was.

At one point he even started to gravity-feed me my liquid food. Gravity feeding is faster than the metered automatic machine because my prescribed liquid protein drink could be measured out and literally poured into a funnel that was attached to the feeding tube in my stomach. The machine I had used previously was very slow and I was missing half of my physical therapy sessions. My dad asked the nurse about this. She said that as long as I could digest the food by gravity feeding and did not get sick or throw up, that would be fine to do, so that's what he did. I never missed my physical therapy again.

He also made sure I had all the proper medications. Whenever I started acting badly or had a reaction, he notified the head nurse and had the medication changed. On two occasions I'd had stitches in my head—once when I arrived without my skull bones and once for two weeks after my skull bones were put back into place. This caused a problem with my having the tendency to scratch the itchy sutures on my head, especially when I first arrived without my skull bones, or flaps, as the doctors called it.

My dad did not want to take the chance that my hand would go up and hit my own head without the skull bones being there, or scratch around the stitches and maybe cause an infection, so he tied my left wrist to the bed frame with a firefighter's safety knot, which quickly would pull apart in an emergency by simply pulling one end of the cotton strap; and he tied the other hand to his right hand when I slept. Tying my hand to his hand was helpful. This prevented me from scratching or accidentally banging my head; his arm would be pulled whenever I tried to reach for my head. The last thing my dad wanted was for me to cause any additional damage.

At first the doctors on staff were very encouraged that my dad was so proactive. But as time went on they weren't so pleased with my dad during my stay at A.I. duPont Hospital. He always made sure I had the right medications and wouldn't hesitate to say something if I wasn't responding well to the medications. He fought for my best interests. For example, I didn't have a wheelchair that fit my body properly. The hospital only had wheelchairs for younger patients, and the wheelchair I'd been given forced my back to stay straight. However, my back had a natural curve, or scoliosis, from years of bad posture and a quick growth spurt. This particular chair did have a curve allowing one to lean back, but this chair forced my back in the opposite direction, forcing me to sit straight. The hospital staff believed that I had back problems from the car accident. My dad had to prove to them with medical records that I had scoliosis prior to my accident.

It also took the longest time for me to get an AFO (ankle, foot orthosis), a foot brace that would help me keep my legs stiff and straight to stand. Years later, I came in contact with my former nurse, Mary. She told me that my dad's constantly bringing irregularities to the doctor's attention and sticking his nose in to make sure everything was right made a difference for the hospital. Now when they have weekly parent "Team Meetings" with the therapists and doctors, a poster-size check-off list is on the wall, making sure that all of the parents' requests are spoken about and followed through on, to the parents' satisfaction.

Once I had the surgery to put in my skull bone flaps, I had protection for my brain and was able to function better. This operation is called a bilateral cranioplasty, obviously because I had both sides removed. I don't know if it was because my brain felt protected, but I started getting better mentally and was becoming more familiar with my surroundings. It was kind of like turning on a light switch or rebooting a computer.

In a matter of weeks, I started to improve tremendously. Therapists and others were happy and surprised. When a person has brain surgery and their entire skull or pieces are removed to heal the brain from the swelling, don't be completely discouraged that the patient isn't doing much. Do know that when the pieces of the skull are placed back over the patient's brain, life can be new and confusing.

One night I got scared and I yelled at my dad sleeping on the bed next to me and said, "Who the *hell* are you?"

He said, "I'm your father."

I replied, "No, you're not!"

He replied, "What do you think, I'm a hired hand?"

I responded, "Yes!"

He said, "Do you think a hired hand would be here twenty-four hours a day, seven days a week? Evan, I'm your father. You were in an accident. You are in a hospital. You are safe."

I found out later that my dad said that to me every day, all the time. He said it so often that at one point I had to ask him to stop it. It ended up being four months before I remembered who my father was. For some reason, I remembered my best friend Ricardo and my mom first.

There was one day after my skull pieces were put back into place that my motivational drive from sports was alive again. I saw a nine-year-old girl in rehab starting to walk with assistance while I was still in a wheelchair. I told my dad, "I want to do that!" I was jealous; here I was, seventeen years old and the captain of my swim team. I should have been walking, not sitting in a wheelchair.

I was so excited for physical therapy the next day. I asked my dad almost every ten minutes, "When is PT?" I asked so often because my immediate memory was awful. With my car accident, I had damaged the front and right side of my brain; my memory was damaged and my brain was still trying to reroute itself and find new circuits. Calmly, he kept responding, "It's at one o'clock."

Finally it was time for PT. I boldly said to my physical therapist Nicole, "I want to walk!" She replied, "Well, Evan, when you get stronger, we can try it. I'm not sure if you're ready yet. Eventually you will be, though." I wasn't too fond of her response, so I said, "No! I want to walk now!" I stood up with her assistance, holding onto an adult-size walker with grip handles for a few seconds. I was ecstatic that I was standing next to the two-foot raised mat platform for a period of time instead of lying down on the platform. My dad said my legs shook like a jackrabbit, but I almost refused to sit down I was so happy.

My Uncle Sam came to see me every day during his lunch break. He always joked around that I was eating mush food. Since I hadn't yet relearned how to swallow, my food was pureed so I could swallow it. I had to do a special swallow test to see if my brain would know how to work the tongue movement to be able to swallow. They sat me up next to a live x-ray machine and my speech therapist fed me a very small amount of different textured foods, kind of like a little taste. She then examined if the proper movement was happening in order for me to swallow. She said that I passed the swallow test based on her observations. This might sound simple, but this was a major hurdle to be able to take in real food, even if it was "mush." Mush was very good, compared to ingesting food through a tube coming out of my stomach.

My speech therapist, Samantha, wanted to know if I'd like to take part in a video that would be used for college students who were studying speech therapy. This was proposed because they'd never seen someone heal as fast as I had from an injury as severe as mine, and they rarely had an older teenager who could talk, as usually the patients were small toddlers. I told her I would do it, but only if I could have a hamburger. She said "Sorry, Evan, I can't do that." Firmly, I replied, "Then I can't do a video." I really didn't want to be videotaped in the state that I was in, so I just let the students sit in on some of my therapy sessions. I didn't get a hamburger until I was ready, a few weeks later. I had to be able to eat pureed food, then semi-pureed food, and finally solid food.

I hated group therapy. It seemed like a waste of time, having to be with other patients and talk about our lives, the reason we were in the hospital, and so on, so we could all bond. I was more focused on getting better so I could leave the hospital. After a while, I was sick of it and felt I'd rather be in the hospital-provided school learning and not part of a group therapy where everyone would just keep expressing our feelings to other patients. It is hard to be happy when you are mentally and physically challenged from an injury. I can see maybe talking about it once or twice, but why dwell on it and always discuss the same thing? Possibly this was to remind the patients of the problem, in case their memory was damaged.

Yes, I can see that I was in a way wrong for not wanting to hear everyone's problems. It's good to be social and engage with other patients who are going through struggles similar to your own. I just felt I was at the healing stage where I wanted to spend more time in school and get back to where I was. The two psychologists weren't pleased with this and it didn't lighten any tension between the doctors and my dad.

When I began to text again, I didn't have a filter to know exactly what I was saying to my guy friends and female friends. After I got my hands on my phone, I looked through my contacts for girls' names. I found six girls and texted them, including an ex-girlfriend from the previous year. I tried to smooth talk those girls, but I actually wasn't that smooth when talking to them. Since I had nothing better to do and no worries in the world, I was obsessive and very forward and I did not make clear sense in my texts.

My communication skills with these girls didn't end well, but since I was severely injured I am hoping they all understood. Honestly, those girls were more excited to see that I was okay than to start an intimate relationship with me.

If you are a friend, parent, or close to someone who is in the hospital and had brain trauma or any kind of injury that hurts their ability to communicate and they start texting again, here is some advice. Warn the people the patient is texting or talking to not to hold anything against him or her, because the patient may not have a filter and they are likely to say anything, whether it's appropriate or not. It is good, however, to start communicating with peers again. It can make the patient feel they are getting back to their normal life.

My relationships with nurses were, I guess you could say, flirty. I hit on almost every nurse, some of whom were pregnant. I would relentlessly tell them to name their baby Evan. No one did. In the beginning of my hospital stay, when I couldn't communicate, I pinched nurses wherever and whenever I could reach. They later told me that I had the strongest grip and it was very painful. One time, my Uncle Sam was near me and I decided to feel his fingers. I noticed that he was wearing a ring. I gripped on the ring so hard that I actually bent and broke it. This awkward, inappropriate behavior is normal with a traumatic brain injury. Thank God it only lasted for about a week. From what I have learned, sometimes patients get stuck in this mode and never come out of it and act inappropriately for the rest of their lives.

# Chapter Four
## *Coming Home*

*Nothing can stop the man with the right*
*mental attitude*
*from achieving his goals; nothing on earth*
*can help*
*the man with the wrong mental attitude.*
*—Thomas Jefferson*

My parents had a decision to make for me. Should I graduate high school or repeat twelfth grade? I had passed all my classes and I technically had enough credits and the grades to pass; I just didn't complete my gym and health classes yet. The school offered to allow me to pass so that I could graduate and be exempt from those two classes. I still was not up to college level, or for that matter twelfth grade level; and if I graduated, then the school district would not have to be responsible for my education. That would mean my parents would have to provide me with the necessary tutoring and education to get me back to a college-prep level. I wouldn't be given the free public education to heal my brain.

Since it was mandatory in the State of New Jersey to take health and gym classes, my parents wanted me to repeat my senior year. It seemed to be the wisest move, both educationally and economically. They told me the scenario and let me make the decision. I told them I would repeat my senior year only if I could swim. My father said he would have to see if I was allowed to swim. He promised me that he would do everything he could to make it possible, so I agreed to repeat my senior year.

I had competed for almost all the eight semesters in high school, except for the last three of my swim meets. Unfortunately, I wasn't allowed to competitively swim for my high school again. My dad had to make a formal request in writing to my high school for them to argue the case to the New Jersey Interscholastic Athletic Association to allow me to swim. My dad also had to have a written statement from my neurosurgeon, Dr. Sugarman, allowing me to swim competitively.

Later that year, the school fought my case with the New Jersey State Interscholastic Athletic Association and we won, allowing me to race the last three meets I had missed from my accident. The NJIAA rarely grants these requests, so this may have been one of the first times that someone has ever won a case for a student to compete in a sport in his fifth year in high school. However, I wasn't physically where I liked or wanted to be, so I decided to not swim. Instead, I focused on my academic recovery in order to reach my goal of going to college in the fall of 2010.

In May of 2009 my dad contacted my high school and requested that I be enrolled in the Special Education Program at Schalick High. In the beginning of June, my high school's Child Study Team came to A.I. duPont Hospital to evaluate me to determine where I was academically and to see where they would place me in the Special Education Program. The Child

Study Team was required to set up an Individual Educational Plan, or IEP, for me. They decided among themselves that my best fit was in a special needs class. This was an appropriate place for a person who had as severe a brain injury as mine.

## Graduating with My Class

My Uncle Sam was telling me I was going to walk for my high school graduation. I had my doubts though. I had six weeks to get stronger and be able to walk with my graduating high school class in '09. At this point, in April, I was barely standing up for five seconds with assistance. I was preparing to go in a wheelchair and asked a few friends if they would push me down the aisle. The school administration preferred to have someone who was not graduating do it instead. However, day by day I became stronger and was able to walk with a walker at the hospital. The therapist aide, Adam, who would often cheer me on, told me, "You're not going in a wheelchair for your graduation. You are walking!" This extra comfort and motivation helped me prepare myself for the big day.

The outdoor graduation day came. The weather wasn't looking good, with occasional showers and rain in the forecast, so the graduation was inside rather than outside. This was actually a blessing for me. I was able to walk with a walker on the smooth gym floor. I chose to walk with Mr. Fortelli, the police officer whose nine-year-old daughter had been severely hurt with a traumatic brain injury and was at A.I. duPont Hospital the same time I was. There were rumors going around, especially with my friends at school: Is Evan going to be at graduation? This was because my mom walked in the graduation practices. I went to the last graduation practice and a good amount of people were surprised and excited to see me.

Graduation day finally arrived. When I first walked into the gym, I was all dressed up in a suit with my cap and gown on, with Officer Fortelli walking beside me. I got the loudest cheers and ovation from the audience, with everyone being totally amazed that I was there; they could hardly believe their eyes. Every time my name was announced or when I went up to get my diploma, there was a standing ovation. There was not a dry eye to be found. My picture was on the front page of all the local and countywide newspapers. Ironically, the class president at the beginning of the year chose *Hope* as the class theme of the graduating class of 2009. Even though I was not actually graduating, only going up with the class I would have graduated with, the day was a great success. I had reached my goal of going to my graduation and walking up with my class.

I found that setting short-term goals with standing and walking helped me get better. If you have an ultimate goal, you stay starved to reach that goal. This time, my ultimate goal was walking at graduation. My next goal was to get myself academically and physically up to par for going to college in the fall of 2010.

## New Home Away from Home

In June I became an outpatient at A.I. duPont Hospital and stayed at the Ronald McDonald House near the hospital. When I first became a member of the Ronald McDonald house, I arrived with a wheelchair, even though I could walk with a walker for a short distance with guidance. The front desk workers always saw me coming with a wheelchair and struggling to get in and out of the car with the wheelchair, with my dad's assistance. Then one day, when I became much better at walking with the walker, the wheelchair wasn't needed at all.

The first time they saw me with a walker, their eyes opened wide in amazement. They were so happy to see me walking and not struggling with a wheelchair. Every morning I went to the hospital for therapy. When I was finished, I enjoyed my stay at the Ronald McDonald House.

My short half-mile car rides from the Ronald McDonald House to the hospital were not very pleasant because my equilibrium was off and I got sick to my stomach. My brain was still trying to reboot itself and regulate all the normal things that people take for granted and do without even thinking about them. My neurons were messed up and still trying to make connections and my body was used to staying stationary. This caused me to have motion sickness whenever I was in a car.

The Ronald McDonald House was a great stay. This house offered more of a roomy atmosphere to live in, compared to the hospital room where I had stayed for more than five months. The Ronald McDonald House offered a nice big room with two king size beds, a TV, bathroom with a shower, and a great food selection for lunch and every night at dinnertime. There was also a PlayStation, a game room, and a gym downstairs, which I enjoyed very much.

As I continued to improve, I refused to quit trying. Maybe because I was a devoted athlete and that athletic mindset was the drive needed to get better. I had been working very hard in my therapy sessions, learning how to walk with my AFO leg braces. One night when my dad and I went down to dinner, I did not want to use my wheelchair or walker. Everyone was amazed to see me up on my own two feet.

Victoria, the social worker at the Ronald McDonald House, was so inspired that she asked us to speak at a fundraising event at a nearby golf course country club, to which the donors of the

Ronald McDonald House had been invited. Here my dad gave a speech on his appreciation of our stay at the Ronald McDonald House.

After our meal and speech at the golf course, Victoria gave us four tickets to see an Eagles pre-season game. Even though I wasn't an Eagles fan, it was nice to see the big premiere of Mike Vick playing with the Eagles. It was nice spending time with my dad at the game and watching football instead of being in a hospital setting. Our seats were all the way up at the top of the upper deck. It was challenging to be able to walk without my walker in the stadium and climb that high, but I was proudly able to accomplish that task.

During the time I lived at A.I. duPont Hospital and the Ronald McDonald House, my parents began to build an addition to our house for me that would be fully accessible and allow me to come home. Eventually, I was on my way home. I was very thankful for the accommodations at the Ronald McDonald House and very excited that I had progressed to the point where I could return home. But this also meant that I had to move on to new places for therapy.

My family lives in South Jersey, about forty minutes from A.I. duPont Hospital, so this wasn't the most ideal or practical place for frequent trips for therapy. My dad had always been very persistent at A.I. duPont Hospital with staying on top of anything I might need. This also seemed to cause tension between my dad and the doctors, because my dad never stopped until I got what I needed for therapy or for the things that would help me get better. Oddly enough, the doctors were the ones who told my dad to be my advocate; now it seemed they didn't want him to be. Anyway, he was my advocate then and still is now.

As tension increased between my dad and the doctors, my dad started locating and interviewing rehabilitation facilities near our home. He found Weisman Rehabilitation Hospital; a good choice for me because the staff had experience with traumatic brain injury (TBI) patients and the hospital was closer to my home. He arranged with the facility to enroll me as an outpatient. Weisman Hospital then made the necessary arrangements with our healthcare provider.

Typically, when a patient is in rehab at a hospital, the goal is to get you in a position to no longer live at the hospital; to help transition you enough in rehab so you can get on with your life and go home. The philosophy of how a hospital does business is great, and it is in the best interest of both the patient and the hospital. In our case with A.I. duPont Hospital, however, my dad was apparently too much of an advocate for me. I think they wanted my dad out of the hospital more than they wanted me out of rehab. I guess you could say we beat them to the punch. We moved on before they could kick my dad and me out.

Mainly because of scheduling reasons, we were able to give A.I. duPont Hospital only two days' notice that we were leaving them and going to Weisman Rehabilitation facility. Our strategy with our insurance company was set in place to give me the full amount of visits; it's better for the insurance to see the full fifteen visits before going to a new place, rather than fewer, where they would expect you don't need as much therapy anymore. This didn't put the therapists at A.I. duPont Hospital in a good situation, and the psychologists were pretty aggravated. They were already not fond of us when I got out of group therapy and they wanted to meet up again. However, we did what was best for us, and it was time to enter new therapies.

Yes, departing the hospital could have gone more smoothly; but A.I. duPont Hospital did an excellent job building a ladder for my future and a successful recovery and good outcome.

# Chapter Five
## *Religion*

*When we are no longer able to change a situation,*
*we are challenged to change ourselves.*
*—Viktor E. Frankl*

After my car accident, I was confused on what happened. I didn't really think, "Why did this happen to me? I'm a good person." I didn't want to think too much about the past regarding my accident. It happened, and there was nothing I could do to change the situation. The only thing I could do was get better.

Before my car accident, I had attended a Christian church with my mom. It was nice, but I didn't have a serious relationship with God. I was just going with the flow and believing in God, while living my life doing the right things.

When pastors came to visit me in the hospital, I listened to what they had to preach. I kept giving myself credit to be where I was in recovery, due to my motivation. However, I could only do so much; being treated in the ICU, I had to give credit and appreciation to the doctor, his assistants, and, ultimately, God. If you have faith and believe in a higher being, that's all that matters. And if you don't believe in God or a higher being that's okay too. Just go based on what you believe and let people go about their own lives, and maybe someday that atheist might be more intrigued to learn about God.

My mother is a Jew who believes in Jesus Christ. Ironically, my neurosurgeon, Dr. Sugarman, is an Orthodox Jew. When I saw Dr. Sugarman a few months later and my dad told him that my mother was Jewish, all of a sudden Dr. Sugarman became excited and said, "Oh, then you're Jewish too!" You see, when the mother is Jewish, her children are automatically considered Jewish.

## Catholicism

The following is a reflection from the priest who anointed and blessed me while I lay at Christiana Hospital in critical condition.

> Entering the room, I could see Evan was hooked up to all sorts of machines. It scared the living daylights out of me and gave me that terrible feeling in the pit of my stomach for Evan's family. But I could also feel the presence of God in the room; it was clear to me He was there and in a powerful way.
>
> As I began to administer the sacrament, God's presence intensified. It's hard for me to put into words; it is the feeling you get deep down inside, one of love and hope, the voice of God stirring in your soul. When I was done with the sacrament of the sick, I held Evan's hand and prayed. I could see all his family watching me with very intense and desperate looks. I prayed, "Lord, save the boy. Heal him and return him to these good people so that they may see your power and glory and your love." As soon as I finished, I heard a voice in my mind that said, "Not only will he be healed, but you will see him walk towards you!" I was shaken by the voice; it had been as clear as daylight. I looked back at the family, and the

voice said, "Tell them." But I doubted in that moment, thinking, *What if it was my own wishful thinking and I tell this family something so specific and he dies later?* I am ashamed I did not speak up, but God was good to me in His patience. I did tell them, "I think he will be okay." I said that because, when I was praying holding his hand, Evan squeezed my hand back, and tightly, especially when I said to him, "I am praying for you."

Eventually Evan began to heal, and here is where the story begins to come full circle. I was ministering at St. Anne's in Elmer at the time where Sam, Evan's uncle, attended Church. Sam told me that Evan wanted to attend mass. So, one faithful Saturday evening, there was Evan, at church and looking better. The whole parish was excited. The prophetic words I had ignored would soon become a reality. During Mass just before we begin the Eucharistic prayer, we have the presentation of the gifts to the altar. As I walked to the front of the sanctuary, I could see Evan with his family bringing up the gifts, and Evan was first in line. It still didn't hit me until he was just a few feet away; the voice came back and said, "You will see him walk towards you." And not only was he walking towards me, but he was carrying the hosts that would soon be consecrated. I couldn't move; I was stunned. He walked towards me from the back of the church all the way to the Sanctuary and handed me the gifts that would become the Body and Blood of our Lord. It gives me the chills, remembering it all.

I couldn't wait for the end of mass so I could talk to the family. When I was outside greeting them, I was so happy for Evan. He approached me and said, "Father, I would like to complete my sacraments and be a fully initiated Catholic."

Before my car accident, I was told that I once spoke about religion to an uncle who was visiting from Minnesota. I told my uncle that I was interested in a more structured type of religion, because I felt I was just going through the motions. With my Uncle Sam being Catholic, now I had a chance of getting involved with a more structured religion. My dad was more interested in reading the bible and watching bible shows on television. Many churches prayed for me while I was in the hospital, and eventually I visited most of them. Then I had the option to attend Saint Mary's Catholic Church every Saturday night.

After I started going to church with my Uncle Sam, I started to learn about Catholicism from the same priest who blessed me at the hospital. It was interesting learning about the Catholic religion and biblical stories. For the next six months I went with my dad to see the priest twice a month to study the bible and the teachings of Jesus Christ, until the point I had my confirmation ceremony as a Catholic on Easter Sunday. The priest shared some good wisdom regarding attending church and praying. He felt that a person shouldn't go to church just to sing and feel happy; the purpose of going to church was to hear the pastor or priest preach and to try to live that way the other six days of the week.

Now I try to pray and reflect on life every night. Faith is a choice; feel free to follow the path you choose. Sometimes when you go through a tragic time, it strengthens your relationship with God.

## Reset Button

When I went back to high school, I needed an aide to walk with me at school, because my balance and coordination were off and my body was still weak. My aide was the 24-year-old teacher and basketball coach. I was relieved that he was my aide. It was bad enough I had to repeat my senior year when a lot of my friends were off to college.

His name was Kirk, and we had a lot in common. We both liked sports and, more importantly, we were both Washington Redskins fans! I was surprised he was a Redskins fan like me, considering neither of us lived in that team's area. He told me he grew up a Redskins fan, because his uncle was a Redskins fan. Since I grew up in northern California, I had started out a fan of the San Francisco 49ers. Unfortunately, it was difficult for me to watch any 49ers games while living in New Jersey. My cousin's husband got a job working for the Redskins and I was able to go to some games, so I started following and rooting for the Redskins. On the bright side, I would be able to see more games, with me living in an area that had a team in the same division.

The first day of school was rough, interesting, and overwhelming. Prior to that first day, my mindset wasn't the greatest: I wasn't pleased that I was going back to high school when I should be swimming for a college. Also, a lot of my friends were no longer students at this high school. It wasn't a happy day to return there. When I walked down the hallways, teachers and students would notice me and say hi; and they seemed excited to talk to me. This continued for about a month or two. It was exhausting, especially since I wasn't thrilled returning to my high school, but I knew they were glad for my recovery. The constant presence of Kirk made school easier.

Before school started, I figured that I would be in special education classes, since I had summer tutoring, also known as extended school year tutoring with the Child Study Team. However, I was in for a surprise. This was my first day in special needs class.

When changing classes, I preferred to get right to my classroom and not be in the hallway seeing peers and other teachers, since I wasn't happy having to repeat twelfth grade. When I arrived in my classroom, my mindset was to be focused and get this day over with. My classmates came into class and things seemed okay. Some students were goofy and immature, but nothing to be concerned about.

Once we started doing schoolwork, though, I became concerned. The first day we did basic elementary schoolwork. I thought to myself, *Okay, this is the first day. Maybe the teacher is just trying to get her students back in the mindset of being back to school and starting off with something easy.* This continued the next few days, so finally I spoke with my teacher and said I feel that I am past this educational level, and she agreed. She was concerned, wondering if this special needs class would be appropriate for me. After she discussed my situation with the Child Study Team, they felt it wouldn't be good to hold me back from progressing.

When someone has had as serious an injury as I'd had, it's common to be relearning life skills. People heal at different rates, and there is nothing wrong with that. As long as the person continues to try to progress, things will fall into place.

At first the decision was made for me to be placed in a regular Algebra 2 and English class. I tried, but these classes moved a little too fast. It was hard to remember what I had learned in class, and my grades showed it. Being concerned about my GPA, I wanted to let the Child Study Team know I was struggling in classes and wanted to explore a better alternative.

We decided to do school tutoring that covered a broader version of English and math. My tutors were Kirk and Mrs. Long. Mrs. Long tutored me at the end of the summer in August, before

I repeated the twelfth grade, so I was comfortable with her. A plus side for me was she taught at the local community college. This seemed to be more appropriate, and it made me feel more comfortable and confident about repeating my senior year. I'd have at least a little connection with college. Mrs. Long taught me English on Mondays, Wednesdays, and Fridays. Kirk taught me math on Tuesdays and Thursdays and was my aide when I walked in the halls every day.

Every week as the school year passed through the fall and spring semester, I was getting better physically and mentally. I was doing more advanced math and English as time went by, to prepare me for college.

The whole reason I was repeating twelfth grade was because I didn't take the senior gym and health class, which is a New Jersey state requirement. Originally the plan was for me to be in a special needs class and take gym and health with them. My gym class was with the special needs class and the part-time vocational students who had a school schedule; that fit perfectly, to have the latest gym class. Honestly, I felt awkward and out of place with this gym class in the beginning. In the past, I'd become accustomed to being with my friends. Eventually, though, I felt more comfortable with the two diverse groups of students. This is a natural feeling for anyone, whether you had a brain injury or not. When entering a new environment, it takes time for the changes to feel more comfortable.

My relationship with the special needs students and vocational students got better as time went on. I was still limited physically in what I could do. Since I was unable to run, I had poor balance, and my coordination wasn't good, this didn't put me in a good situation for competing well with my classmates. Before my accident I had been athletic and able to excel in the gym games. Compared to that, my not being able to physically compete was discouraging and embarrassing. I accepted my limitations quickly, though, and went about my business communicating with my classmates. Games I participated in were mostly walking the track and playing tennis and basketball. These activities helped me work on my individual goal of gradually getting better physically.

The special needs students established a strong bond with me. At the end of the school year, they made a thoughtful "Good Luck in College!" card for me. Their teacher took me aside and said, "I don't really say this often, but the way the kids look up to you and engage with you, I feel you have the gift of being a special needs teacher. Some people naturally have it." I thought that was a nice compliment, but being a teacher had never interested me as a career.

After a year had passed since my car accident, I was introduced to a new lifestyle at school and at home: I was no longer as independent as I had been in the past. Having to adapt to a lifestyle where I was dependent on my family and the unique new high school experience actually helped me mature into a young adult. I was nicer and more empathetic to my family and peers.

I saw my friend Dan once or twice that year, and he was shocked to see me—not only because I was alive, walking and talking, but also because of other things he observed, like how I communicated! Every time we talked, I actually seemed to care about what he was saying. This surprised him as completely as had my miraculous recovery. Also, he said I looked very determined. I wasn't able to walk well, but I wanted to be independent while standing and walking. I became irritated if my parents came close to give me guidance.

My mom told me a funny story about my wanting to walk independently. In the summer, before I repeated my last year in high school, I kind of made a scene while shopping in Rite Aid. My mom said, "I was following you intently to make sure you didn't trip or fall while you were walking." But she said I was getting annoyed, wanting to have my own space, so she reluctantly allowed me. Shortly after that, there was a noise! When she looked around the corner, she chuckled and said "My, my, my. Look at you, Evan." I was covered in boxes from the display in between the aisles. I shook my head, looked at her, and then replied with a laugh, "I learned my lesson!"

The year I was still in high school I was allowed to skip my last period. But my day wouldn't be over to relax. Instead, I would go to all of my therapies. The first therapy place I went to was Weisman Center for physical and speech therapy. In my physical therapy, one of the unique exercises we tried was to stop my "dropped foot" motions in my right foot. Something like this is common for a person who has had brain trauma, because the person's neurons are damaged and it can trigger limitations throughout the body.

My physical therapist taped my right foot and calf with electrifying motion detectors that shocked me if I wasn't walking smoothly. This was a neat product that gave me awareness if I was walking with a dropped foot. In order to heal "drop foot," a person needs to be aware that they are doing it. Getting your ankle stronger is important. To strengthen my ankle, I used an elastic band to bring my foot up and down. Another therapy I had at Weisman was aquatic therapy. I was excited to do this therapy, because I still had a strong desire to swim.

## Initial Outpatient Rehabs

Weisman Children's Hospital opened a new rehab facility and not a lot of people were familiar with the added location. Weisman is a well-established hospital in central Jersey, where they treat children, as does A.I. duPont Hospital. When I first started my rehab, it was refreshing not seeing many patients that were younger than me, although Weisman Center became more popular as time passed, bringing more children to the rehab center. My dad and I noticed this, and we felt it would be appropriate to begin a search for a new rehab location, even though the physical and speech therapies were good.

At Weisman, my initial speech therapist was good. Yes, I did some kids' memory games, but she tried to make it as age appropriate as possible. Once she even had me read an article in my ESPN magazine and remember the specifics of what was said in the article. Unfortunately, she was pregnant and went on maternity leave and would permanently leave that Weisman location while I was still a patient there.

Speech therapists at the outpatient Weisman Center usually treat children. The first therapist to treat me after my original therapist left had me do children's memory games, and then she ran out of things to do. She said, "Want to read Barney?"

I responded "No." And my therapy that day was finished. I immediately told my dad, and he said yes, it was time to move to a new therapy. After that incident, he wasted no time in starting to look for new rehab facilities.

My dad found a place for me to do physical and speech therapy: HealthSouth Rehabilitation Hospital. These hospitals are built for adult patients, and I had turned eighteen a few months prior. Finally! I was able to start doing rehab in a place where I wasn't surrounded by children.

I immediately felt this therapy was more age appropriate for me, now that I was an adult. An important thing my dad did was to get legal guardianship for me so that he could still make decisions for me and get me into the different rehabilitation facilities and legally inquire and ask questions on my behalf.

Right from the beginning, I liked my speech therapy more than my previous stints. In my speech therapies at A.I. duPont Hospital and Weisman, speech therapy was oriented to kids. During my speech therapy at HealthSouth, I read and comprehended articles that were better suited to my age.

The physical therapy was a conservative approach. I mostly walked on the treadmill, did legs equipment lifting, and did balancing exercises. My physical therapist started to shorten my visits to the insurance company, making it look like I was getting "all better," and that she was such a great physical therapist. My dad demanded that the report be amended and additional therapies be added. To the surprise of HealthSouth, the insurance company granted the additional sessions. My dad had always been in direct contact with the insurance company's utilization management department. They were fully aware of my continued progress and miraculous ongoing recovery, so they always granted the therapy for me. My dad always said it was not him that made it happen; it was God and divine intervention.

After these incidents of trying to lower my visits and get me out of rehab, my dad once again started to look for a new facility. We changed places again. This time I had speech therapy at Inspira Health Network and physical therapy at Achieve Physical Therapy & Fitness. My therapies continued for the next seven months. I will talk more about those later.

# Chapter Six
## *Competitive Edge*

*The principle is competing against
yourself. It's about self-improvement,
about being better than you were the day
before.*
*—Steve Young*

Throughout my recovery I was still interested in swimming for my summer league. Our local swim club league has a cutoff age on when a swimmer is allowed to compete. Swimmers are allowed to compete until the age of eighteen, and June is the cutoff month for the swimmer's birthday. Since my birthday was in September, I was able to make the cutoff date and would be eligible to compete. Before the accident, I was excited that I would be able to go to college one year, then come back and competitively swim.

However, things didn't turn out as planned. I went back and completed twelfth grade instead of attending my first year at college. I don't say this out of regret because I never complained about it. I just set my goals and stayed focused on the positive things I wanted to accomplish. In swimming, I wanted to get a lot faster and to be able to dive off a block to race again. My physical ability was very limited.

I remember in the fall I joined fall warm-ups like I always had in the past with Ricardo. I was with people our age, and it was all right. I swam in the slower lane in practice, and I felt okay with it. During this time of my recovery I was unable to dive off the block. When I went to training practice with Ricardo it was okay. The instructors were more concerned with getting our endurance back up in the pool. Overall, I was dissatisfied with my swimming speed; I was a little intimidated by how fast the swimmers were practicing in the pool, and I couldn't keep up. I was optimistic, though, because I had months to get physically more prepared and faster in the pool for the summer. That's how it went in the beginning of my recovery and first swimming training sessions. Now I had a real challenge in front of me.

Springtime had come. I had been working hard on getting my legs stronger and more coordinated. I even got to the point of beginning to hop a few inches. But the time was here. Get prepared for the summer swimming league.

Earlier in the spring, realizing that summer was getting closer, I joined spring swimming warm-ups at a different location, compared to the fall training. I was attracted to these spring warm-ups because of how they were described: Their signups were labeled something along the lines of a technique and fine-tuning swimming program. Plus these swimmers were probably not as fast as the other swimmers I swam with in the fall. This was good. I was always concerned with the smoothness I had with my swimming strokes in the pool. The car accident had damaged my ability to swim backstroke and freestyle. If I could correct these swimming mechanics errors, then I'd be able to swim effectively in the summer.

The first day I was excited to get back in the pool and train for my summer team. I told a few of my friends, the teacher aide Kirk, and my physical therapist about my swimming plans. I entered the pool and saw a bunch of swimmers ages nine through fourteen. My heart sank. Yes, the age range for this program was ten through eighteen, but I was expecting the older swimmers to be separated from the younger ones. That was not the case. I hated going to every single practice for those six weeks.

That spring, swim warm-ups didn't represent a happy time in my life. It was even more depressing that a few of these children were faster than me. I mean, some of them were really fast. One of the swimmers asked how old I was. I replied, "Eighteen."

Surprised, he said, "No, you're sixteen."

I corrected him and said that I was eighteen. Eventually I got aggravated and said, "Yeah, I'm sixteen." There was this tiny Asian nine-year-old who was pretty much a swimming phenom. He passed me in the pool often, which was even more depressing.

I did get some good strengthening exercise in this spring warm-up, though. My legs were getting stronger and my coordination was improving. After telling the coach about my traumatic brain injury, he helped me step onto the block and dive. This was rewarding because I knew I was close to my goal, racing for my summer team.

My swimming strokes, flip-turns, and endurance improved. When I was at practice, I noticed that some of the kids liked to single out and pick on one younger, smaller and faster swimmer, sometimes because of his race. That swimmer, who was picked on, was very encouraging and rooted for me, especially when I was struggling to dive off the block. Later his mom came up to me and said, "My son was excited to see there's a new swimmer and he knew you were intelligent, because the coaches never talked back to you."

I don't think the coaches would have even considered saying anything negative to me, with my unique circumstances, as I occasionally stood at the end of the pool to catch a breather while the other swimmers kept practicing. She told me that her son was having problems with the other kids picking on him and the coaches didn't like him being so fast, more mature and of a different race. I never saw him again because I skipped the last two practices, thinking I'd had enough and my summer team was starting up soon.

I began to dislike swimming and became less interested in the sport because of the embarrassing experiences. I reached a point where I wasn't looking forward to the summer league. With fear and dread, I didn't even want to count down the days for the swim team to start again.

## Achieving My Goals!

In the spring, after I was done with HealthSouth, we needed to find a new therapy place for me. Every rehab place I had ever gone to in the past was run by a hospital. Generally, a rehab in the hospital has a more conservative approach to physical therapy. A self-owned therapy place is freer to use more advanced and challenging exercises to enhance the patient's improvement. My mom works as a massage therapist at a hospital and gym. Her boss was mentioning a sports rehab place that he knew had done a great job in the past for athletes.

My dad visited the recommended therapy place I mentioned earlier, Achieve Physical Therapy & Fitness. When he checked out the rehab place, he spoke to a therapist, George. Ironically, George happened to have been my soccer coach when I was nine. He vaguely remembered me and ended up being my physical therapist. This was cool. I was excited to try a sports rehab place that would be more aggressive and help me get better physically and reach my goal to competitively swim that summer. Because I was still weak and my balance and coordination were awful, the main goal throughout my rehab was to get stronger and increase my coordination. I did exercises I had tried in the past, plus new, unique ones.

Some other new exercises I started to do were to lie on my stomach and reach, to use the elliptical bike, and to use the floor ladder steps. As I had predicted, George was accommodating to the fact that swimming was only months away. He had me walk in between blocks, balance sitting on a ball, and lastly, at my request, work on my jumping. Jogging on the elliptical really helped my coordination with getting used to the jogging motion and endurance. Using the stationary bike also helped my legs simulate running motions.

Since Achieve was a sports rehab place, they didn't offer anything besides physical therapy. My mom happened to know a guy who was a speech therapist at the hospital where she works. I was interested in having a male therapist, because I was so used to having a female as my speech therapist. He seemed cool, was interested in sports, and was a big talker, preaching how he could really help me. I was very excited doing therapy at my sports therapy place and the speech therapist seemed good.

The speech therapist was very busy; he did therapy at an outpatient rehab center and saw patients in the hospital. But he was confident he could fit me in. Since he knew my mom and wanted to help me, he made an exception for me.

We did similar types of exercises for speech therapy. This was memory from reading, recalling stories I heard, and testing for logic. Even though we were doing what I usually did in therapy, I was happy with him, especially because we talked sports. This lasted for a month or two, but his schedule became too hectic; so we switched to a new therapy place within the same hospital.

With my new therapist it went all right. I told her I was interested in becoming a speech therapist. The reason I was thinking about doing this was that I had the impression it was easy. Having been a patient for speech therapy, I felt it couldn't be that difficult to play memory games with the patient. No big deal, right? She let me shadow her working with a child, to show me it wasn't that easy. The child was unfocused, not obeying her and running everywhere, and that led to problems. That experience quickly changed my interest in speech therapy as a career.

We were told by my high school child study group coordinator and Mrs. Long, one of my high school tutors, about the Department of Vocational Rehabilitation, an agency which helps with funding for people who are disabled. Since I had every intention of going to college, they were considering funding my books and room and board. In order for them to sponsor me, I had to go through a testing at an adult brain injury rehab place. This was a grueling three-day, six-hour-a-day testing. I struggled in some of their tests, such as bookkeeping receipts, neurological testing, and other neurological challenges. I'm not sure how this is related to how successful you will be in college, but one thing I struggled with was a memory game. I guess they want to make sure I could take care of myself on my own. I had to remember twenty words and repeat them in order, remember ten new words and repeat them; and, finally, thirty minutes later, recite the first 20 words that were said.

After all the testing I did with writing, bookkeeping, housekeeping and an overload of other tasks, the doctor, who was the head psychiatrist there, felt I wasn't college-ready. Right before we went into this meeting, my dad had asked me if I wanted to go to college. I said yes. Then my dad said not to worry about what they said, that he and my mom would help pay for the books and room and board. "If you want to go to college, we'll help pay to have you go."

The doctors at the rehab facility told the Department of Vocational Rehabilitation that they would not recommend a full load at college; perhaps three credits at a community college. But my parents had faith in me, and my dad called the counselor in charge and said I would be successful in college. In the end, the Department of Vocational Rehabilitation sponsored me.

## Just Keep Swimming!

The summer swimming season finally arrived, but I wasn't that enthusiastic after my poor showing and discouraging experience in spring warm-ups. My confidence in the pool was shattered after swimming with nine to thirteen year olds, some of whom were faster than me. I went into the lane with my friends, which was the fastest lane. This was the lane I swam in for years. I was exhausted, got passed many times and took breaks, but all in all it was okay. I was more comfortable being passed by people I'd grown up with rather than people at least five years younger than me.

Since my depth perception wasn't great and my brain was only a-year-and-a-half healed, my flip turns weren't consistently good, barely touching the wall with my feet and getting dizzy from the flipping motion. I was advised to just touch the wall with my hand and push off to save time. I was going to physical therapy less often, being exhausted from swimming practices.

My balance and leg strength weren't great, so I needed assistance to get onto the diving block in practice and before races. My swimming friends helped me stand up on the block, and I was grateful; but it got redundant and I felt bothersome, always asking for assistance.

My first swim meet had finally come. I was excited to be racing again. However, my nerves were getting to me, wondering how fast I'd swim, and hoping not to make any mistakes on my flip-turns or getting on the block and diving. This was an unusual emotion to have, considering I'd been so accustomed to competitive swimming, but I had to keep reminding myself times had changed.

In my first meet, I individually swam freestyle and backstroke. I also swam in the B relays, which was now appropriate, not being as fast as I was in the past. As my first race came, I was helped onto the diving block. Some of the parents cheered, being happy to see me swimming again! Being a competitive athlete, I wasn't pleased with my time. But my parents and other parents and friends said, "It is okay. You were able to dive off the block and race again. That's incredible considering where you came from in such a short time period. You finished! There were some swimmers who didn't finish the race." I just nodded my head, but internally I was still frustrated because I was used to swimming faster.

My best stroke, the backstroke, wasn't much better. Though it was nice, not having to be helped on the block to start the race, my coordination was so off! I couldn't swim straight. I kept on drifting to the left side, with my right arm being stronger than my left arm. The race was fifty meters, but since I was drifting so much, I probably swam sixty-five meters. When you swim backstroke, you're forced to do a flip turn after you finish the first lap. In backstroke you have to flip your arm and move to your belly and do a flip turn; then, after the flip, go back into the backstroke position. My problem was flipping too soon because of bad depth perception and the fear of hitting my head. As a result, I'd barely touch the wall or I'd miss it completely. This slowed me down and really put me out of contention from winning.

Since this was the summer league, the team was more laid back compared to the winter league. We had fun activities to do, and it was good to continue to have fun in my chosen sport. Since this was more of a laid back season, I had fun with my peers and sometimes didn't make the most appropriate remarks. A person with brain trauma can behave like this, not having a filter.

I was unable to physically participate in some activities, but I got over it and it was okay. Whenever you're recovering from an injury in the hospital or at home and you're unable to do some activities that you used to be able to do without even thinking about it, it can be frustrating. Just hang in there and keep trying. It's a good test on how you handle tough times. For example, I was practicing my swimming laps with much younger swimmers, and that can be hard emotionally. But the more you persevere, the happier you'll be. My swim times got better throughout the summer, but I'd always finish second to last or last. Still, I had a great time swimming with my team that season, which surprised me after being discouraged in the spring and even though I wasn't fast.

# Chapter Seven
# The Beginning of
# Higher Education Struggles

*In school, you're taught a lesson and then*
*given a test. In life,*
*you're given a test that teaches you a*
*lesson.*
*—Tom Bodett*

I was off to King's College, a Catholic college. I had officially become a Catholic earlier that year of my own free will. Before my accident I had been accepted to this college with an interest in swimming for them. After the college learned about my car accident, the staff prayed for me. The college also kindly held all of my grants and scholarships for the following year, 2010. I was feeling nervous and uncertain about how well I'd do in my college courses. On one hand, I had reached my goal of getting to college. But now, here I was taking college-level courses. This was not the same as being tutored in a mellow high school setting. Since I was part of the Academic Skills Program, I met with Mrs. Smith, the program coordinator, three times a week for the first semester. Her role was similar to that of a guidance counselor or to the role of the special education coordinator in high school. She made sure students were doing okay with all their classes, as well as assisting and teaching us how to manage our time and become fully independent.

When I had tests, I took them at the Academic Skills office. This was a separate, quiet classroom for students who needed extra time for testing. In this Academic Skills office, they had a person who managed tutoring services. At King's College, all students were allowed to receive tutoring for any course, at no charge. It's great that they offer this to help students do well academically. It is uncommon for a college to offer free tutoring for all students in almost any class.

Starting college, I didn't have the best mindset. I thought it was an excuse that I had a traumatic brain injury and it was okay if I didn't do well, or maybe allowed myself to think that. This thought process gave me less motivation to succeed in my classes. That is an awful approach to college! I had been trying so hard to relearn how to do everything in my life again except just learning how to go out and have some fun with friends, so this had me caring more about my social life and the "college experience" and less about college classes and test scores.

The past year and a half I hadn't had much of a social life, being sheltered at my house and not free to be around many peers, most of whom had been away at college. So naturally I was anxious to have fun and embrace my new freedom. For freshmen, teachers are required to send home mid-term grades. To start off, I didn't do my writing homework because I didn't understand how to access the college website and do my homework. For my accounting and algebra classes, I didn't spend enough time studying. That really hurt my test grades and set me back.

When I prioritized my time to social life, I made a lot of friends and acquaintances. Some hobbies I had at college were weightlifting and exercising at the college gym, which I needed to help me get stronger. Before I started attending college, I had joined a Facebook group called King's 2014. This group allowed future students to meet their peers before the semester began. I met Tyrone and ended up being the closest to him for the rest of my stay at college. He was interested in and knowledgeable about lifting. This was helpful, because he gave me some good fitness tips. Since I spent a lot of time lifting, my family was shocked to see me bigger and stronger a month later.

Another hobby I had, other than just hanging out with friends, was playing ping pong. I played ping pong for hours almost every day with Tyrone, Anthony, Fred, and some other friends. This was always fun and competitive, but it took time away from why I was there in the first place: to concentrate on my academics.

Girls! That's what was on my mind when I first got to college. When I was home recovering, I was secluded and didn't have the opportunity to interact with girls I wanted to date. Though I was interested. So, naturally, I was excited and looked forward to meeting new girls at college! When doing so, I was talkative and friendly, but I was also rusty and inexperienced in how to actually flirt and talk to girls who were interested in me. In fact, there were a few occasions where a girl was interested in me, but I was nervous and did nothing, fearing that I'd fail or say something dumb. In high school, before my accident, I'd had a few girlfriends, but it wasn't serious enough to prepare me for college life.

I lived in an underclassman dorm, and people were immature. This led to always having the normal pranks and incidents relating to inexperience in living away from home. The fire alarm went off at least 10 times a semester, thanks to burning popcorn and smoke bombs. Sometimes this didn't happen at the most convenient time! One time the alarm went off at 3:00 a.m. and I had an accounting test that morning! This was a strange experience because, if I had never been hurt, I probably would have never thought about how difficult it was to get shoes on or get dressed in a hurry to get out of the building. When an alarm goes off, the rule generally is to rush outside. However, I still wasn't that coordinated and didn't move quickly. When walking down the steps, I tried to walk fast while holding onto the railing, but my main focus was to make sure I was safe. During the first fire alarm, before I had ever met my friend Anthony, he thought, *If this kid doesn't hurry up, we're going to die! Hurry up!*

## Getting My Act Together

After seeing my mid-term grades, I was disgusted and needed motivation. I posted a sticky note at the top of my computer, where I'd see it often. On that note I had written the name of the brain injury rehab place that had given me a bad recommendation to the Department of Vocational Rehabilitation; previously, they had advised my family that I wasn't ready for multiple college classes. They said that with the distractions and stress that college life gives students, I'd fail out; plus they felt the types of classes were going to be too difficult for me after such a serious brain injury.

They were right—at least, for the first two months—so I made it my mission to prove them wrong, and that sticky note was the start! If I put my mind to it, I could put forth my best effort and succeed. Having them doubt me was actually a blessing in disguise. If I hadn't experienced that negative putdown a few months prior, I don't know if I'd have had the same drive, the same mindset, to continue college in a successful manner. When you're down, it's easy to give up and listen to others' negative opinions. But, if you energize your struggles with a purpose, it makes it a lot easier to stay focused and determined.

For my accounting class, I used the college's services and got a tutor. But, I didn't understand the accounting concept. This set me behind for the next test, where understanding the material in the beginning of the class was important. Since I had to start from the beginning it was difficult to learn new material at the same time. If you are extremely behind, sometimes it's best to withdraw or drop the class if it's early enough not to hurt your GPA. Withdrawing from that class allowed me to concentrate on my other studies that were falling behind. In the end, it was a good thing. I brought all of my grades up by the end of the semester.

The start of the spring semester was more fun. The roommate I'd had the first semester decided to move in with his friend in another dorm, since his friend's roommate had transferred. I had a single room, and my friends often came to my room to hang out. When you're a freshman and don't have a roommate of choice, the college assigns you a roommate based on a small questionnaire. Whether you'd get a compatible roommate was a hit-or-miss proposition. The college was good, but they weren't the best at picking roommates; most of my friends didn't get along with theirs.

# Bright Lights

The next semester I had some difficult courses to take. It would have been nice if I'd started off on a good note. Unfortunately, that wasn't the case. This time my struggle was finite math, which was a more in-depth algebra class that included algebra, statistics, and graphing. The other classes I took were manageable. With the next-level writing class, I did better with doing my homework and staying on top of things, compared to the first semester. Whenever I wrote papers, I thought they were well-written, even after the teacher revised them, and I would tell a few friends that I was proud of my work. When I got grades back, though, I'd get slapped in the face with a less-than-satisfying grade. This puzzled and angered me. After all, I'd been told it was a well-written essay after she edited it, only to find out that it wasn't as good as it could have been. I thought, *Wasn't it supposed to be all better with my teacher editing it?* Time went on and I tried harder and did better than before.

One day I got an email from the school about a lip-syncing contest. I always wanted to do that, but never had the guts to actually do it. In order to compete in this contest, I needed to think of a song. There were so many songs to choose from and I couldn't figure out which song to pick. My friend Anthony said, "Whenever I come to your room, I always hear you playing the song, 'Build Me Up, Buttercup.' That would be a good song to do, in dedication to your writing teacher. You always say how great a paper you wrote and then don't get a good grade." So I picked that song by the Foundations, since my teacher would always build me up, saying how good this paper looks, and then let me down with the grade.

I had one day to prepare. Since I didn't know all the lyrics I listened to the song numerous times. The next day before the contest, I was really nervous. I got dressed up in a suit and tie like "The Foundations" would. I had one of my friends make sure I looked sharp and my tie was tied correctly. My nerves were on edge, but I wanted to be gutsy as I was at a new school and with a fresh start. He tried to comfort me saying, "Dude, even if you don't get first, it's okay. You have the guts to do this. I wouldn't be brave enough to do this."

Tyrone and three other friends were there to support me. I happened to see my accounting tutor, and she asked, "What are you going to do on the stage?" I responded, "I'll probably just stand up and lip-sync my song." She responded "No. You have to walk around so everyone sees you and you should point to people." The time was here. I stood on stage unprepared and was going to have to "wing it." Many people before me were in groups and used props to make it more interesting for the audience. This didn't give me much hope of winning, since I didn't have props and wasn't prepared.

Right when the song started, here came those nervous jitters again, and my legs began to shake slightly. I didn't know what to do. The beat was playing with no vocals yet, so I started to clap to get the crowd into my skit. I was so unprepared; some of my claps didn't even go with the rhythm in the song. Great. After the first lyric in the song played, I opened my mouth and it was dry. Nerves again. After the first thirty seconds, though, I started getting into the moment.

Then I moved my mouth and gave hand gestures, while walking back and forth to each side of the stage and got the crowed into the song. I made sure to point at the crowd whenever the lyrics came, "I need you, I need you, more than anyone, Darling" and at "Why do you build me up, Buttercup, Baby, just to let me down," I did a surprised facial expression while pointing my fingers up and down. Lastly, when the lyric "I'm attracted to you" was said, I decided to wink and point at all the girls in the front. They responded well to that, as they blew through their fingers to make loud whistles. When I was finished, everyone clapped for me. To say the least, I definitely didn't do a good job! I was reminded by my friends who saw my performance that I was bad, but I wasn't the worst: Someone before me just stood in the center and only moved his mouth— something I had originally planned to do!

## Crunch Time with a Good Distraction

Towards the end of the semester I went to a dance club with a friend. We met some girls who didn't go to my college, so we went with them. Bear in mind that I wasn't that coordinated yet and my legs were still weak. To top it off, I'd never been great at dancing, even before the car accident.

So naturally, I thought that this wasn't a good strategy to meet girls. When we got to the club, my dancing was stiff and not good. Since I'm a guy, maybe it didn't look as awful. With my legs being skinny and weak, they quickly got fatigued from moving around for a long period. We were there for two hours. After all that standing and dancing, I walked out in a way that made me seem extremely drunk; my legs felt like Jell-O, and I almost didn't have the strength to walk to the car.

A few weeks later, after the interesting dancing event, one of the guys I went to the club with told me something I wasn't expecting: that Rochelle, a girl from the other college, thought I was cute and she was interested in me. I was excited, but I didn't know which girl he was referring to. After I saw a picture of the girl who was interested in me, I thought, *Well, she's a little big, but she has a cute face.* Nothing had been working for me with girls, so why not be open-minded. I didn't really have my hopes up, but a few days later we met up and, surprisingly, we had a connection!

If you have trauma to the brain, it can be difficult to handle your emotions. If that's the case, it's okay. Just work on it. Eventually you'll be able to compose yourself in a better manner. I was happy, being more independent, and away from home, although with my brain injury I would get out of control and laugh for a *really* long time. Fortunately, times of uncontrollable laughter were the worst side effects I had to deal with. I have been told that traumatic brain injury, TBI, can leave some people with intense anger and sometimes violent outbursts. Sometimes, while with a few friends in the cafeteria, I would laugh for almost twenty minutes over something funny that was said, or sometimes for no other reason except that I thought of something funny. My friends Tyrone, Anthony, and Fred would just think, *Here we go again. Let him do his thing.*

I was still goofy and I hoped when I dated that I'd be able to compose myself and not look like a fool. When I started to date Rochelle I was able to compose myself. I didn't act goofy or do any uncontrollable laughing. This shocked me, but I was relieved; if I went into a twenty-minute laughing episode, it wouldn't have been good. If I got anything from my relationship with her, it was that, in a way, being with her helped fix my uncontrollable laughter—for the most part, that is.

Sometimes when you want something, it doesn't come at the most opportune time. I met Rochelle the week before finals. I had been struggling with finite math. I scored poorly on all three of my tests and needed to do really well on my finals to pass. Literally, I was failing. This was a nerve-wracking time. I wanted to pass a class that I struggled in, yet at the same time I had the excitement of spending time with a girl. That week, pretty much all I did was spend time with Rochelle and study for my finals when I wasn't with her.

I studied a lot! I went over all of the same practice problems eight times. I had to know the formula and feel more confident with taking the finite-math final. It was a cumulative score, making it important to know the material, and I hadn't done as well earlier in the semester. That seemed to be a trend for me, but this time I wanted to keep the class and not withdraw, as I had done with accounting.

I wanted to feel extremely confident when I took that final, so I went to the teacher's office and reviewed with her for an entire hour before the final. I told her, "Pile me with practice questions." This strategy might have tired someone's brain before they even started. But my thought process was that it needed to be fresh in my mind. Nothing else could be on my mind when taking this final. When I did take the final, I was able to remember some of the formulas immediately because they were fresh in my mind. I ended up passing the class with a *C–*.

Rochelle, the girl I'd started to see, happened to live only forty minutes from my parents. This was awesome, almost meant to be. I'd finally started dating someone in college, after not having the best of luck all school year. And the girl I met lived close to my house.

At this time, I had a wide gap in my skull where the body started to reabsorb the skull bone. Imagine a gap running midline, front to back, about an inch wide in the middle of the top of my head. There was no bone in this area to protect my brain. This needed to be fixed with a prosthetic. If I had taken another blow to my brain in this area, my brain would be unprotected. I planned to have Dr. Sugarman perform an operation and implant a skull prosthetic as soon as I finished school that year. I'd been anticipating this surgery for a long time. That meant I would have to be extra cautious and not get sick. If I got sick, I would have to push back my surgery. That would have been a letdown.

One night, two weeks before the semester had finished, my throat started to get a little sore. I was extremely worried that this would hurt my surgery plans. Immediately, I texted Rochelle and asked, "Are you sick?" That's somewhat unusual, something someone doesn't expect to hear, and very abrupt, but I hadn't told her about my traumatic brain injury yet.

After my experience of getting a lot of attention that was overwhelming during my second senior year of high school, I made a rule: I would only tell someone about my car accident under one of these three circumstances:

1. If they asked, noticing that I walked a little awkwardly.

2. If I had to tell them. Examples were a teacher, tutor or, someone who was spotting me in the gym.

3. If I wanted to tell them, feeling they already liked me for who I am and didn't judge me.

Since I wanted to see if Rochelle liked me for who I was, not giving pity or sympathy, I intentionally hadn't told her about my car accident; I wanted to see if the chemistry was real. Later, come to find out, whenever I told more people in college about the accident, it wasn't a big deal.

She responded to my text that she was confused. I'm sure she was thinking, *Am I sick? Did he not like me?* I told her that the next time I saw her I would explain to her why I wanted to know if she was sick. When I met up with her the next day, I found out she was studying to be a nurse and wanted to treat trauma. This added more of a connection and made me more interested in her, because she was an understanding person. After I explained my planned surgery and how I couldn't take a chance on getting sick, she understood why I was concerned. I went to the nurse's office to get all the medication needed so my sore throat would go away.

# Chapter Eight
## *Under the Knife*

*The loss of love is not nearly as painful as*
*our resistance to accepting it is.*
*—Tigress Luv*

On the day before the surgery, I was nervous, relieved, and excited. I thought about how the doctor would be opening up my skull to see my brain again, and putting a prosthesis in place of my reabsorbing skull bone. Soon the top of my head would be protected and restored. Hopefully, everything would be okay during the surgery. At least this surgery was safer because it was not a life-threatening emergency like before. The morning of my surgery I needed to wake up at 4:00 a.m., to undergo surgery two hours later. When I arrived at the hospital, a weird series of events occurred.

When I started undergoing prep routines for the surgery, my first nurse, who was an older lady, told me it was her first day back. She asked, "Where do you go to school?"

I told her, "I go to King's College."

Suddenly, she started bawling tears of joy. She said, "It's meant to be that you're my first patient after coming back from a leave of absence at work." Her dad had just passed away, and he was a King's College graduate in 1948.

Afterwards I had to have some blood work done. The doctor asked where I was going to school. I responded, "King's College." She said, "Oh, I know that college. I went to Wilkes University, the college next to King's." Oddly enough, this was the same university that Rochelle was attending. After I was finished with the blood work, another doctor, an anesthesiologist, was talking to me about weightlifting. He had a voice that was similar to that of the person who had told me Rochelle was interested in me. All these things seemed more than a coincidence.

I came out of surgery and was placed in a recovery room, and then I was moved to a single ICU room. Surrounding me were uncomfortable wires and clips that were attached all over my body. It was awful. Nurses came into my room every two hours to check my blood or to give me medicine. I had cotton gauze wrapped around my skull to keep the sutures clean and covered for a few days; this was very uncomfortable. All around me were beeping monitors. I also had a drain line from my head that made it uncomfortable to sleep.

After my surgery, I was back to square one. I couldn't walk, as if my balance wasn't bad enough to start with. They put me through occupational therapy, where I had to tie my shoelaces, and physical therapy, where I walked around the hospital hallways.

When I was in the hospital after surgery, I was very happy. The surgery I'd been waiting for was finished; Rochelle visited me and met my dad. It's nice that she came. But to top it off, my grades for the semester were available on the computer. I logged into my college account and I saw that I had good grades and had passed finite math. Wow, that was a relief!

Next, I shared a room with a person who was getting ready for brain surgery. He was a Vietnam veteran who became senile and had short-term memory loss. He gave his negative thoughts about the then-current war in Iraq and Afghanistan. I mentioned Rochelle was in ROTC and wanted to be a nurse in the war. This old vet had some strong feelings about the war. That it wasn't smart to be in the war and that too much politics was involved. He thought the main reason they went to war was so they could make money for big companies and get cheap oil. He said it wasn't worth risking your life for that nonsense.

Lastly, Dr. Sugarman came to see how I was recovering from surgery. He was pleased to see how I was doing after surgery and removed some monitoring wires that were no longer needed. A few days later, I was released from the hospital.

I had completed my first year of college, had the much anticipated surgery to protect my brain, and was dating a girl from college who lived close to my house. Things were looking pretty good.

## Summer Loving

That summer, I took my first summer class and ended up taking summer classes the next two summers as well. I decided to take my first summer class at night; it was a new experience. Half of the students in my class were close to my age, the rest were over thirty. For the first test I took, I didn't prepare myself properly. I thought, *It's community college; this test is going to be a piece of cake.* That wasn't the case. I failed that first test. I wrote a paper about the chapter to bring up my grade and did a better job of preparing for the rest of my tests to do well that semester. It's never good to underestimate something.

The first summer break from college was going pretty well. Rochelle tried to drive to my parents' house every weekend. A few weeks after my surgery, she started to get sick. She had mono. I was concerned, hoping I didn't have mono now that I was recouping from my surgery, so I got a blood test. A few weeks later the results showed that I didn't have it; I'd probably had mono as a child and become immune to it. That was a relief. Last thing I wanted was a setback that would hurt my recovery.

Things were going great. Rochelle continued to come over every weekend and we texted all day, every day. I wasn't sure when and if I should make her my girlfriend, but I was happy how it was going. She wasn't officially a girlfriend yet, but I had strong feelings for her. My Uncle Sam was over and asked about my situation with girls in general. I happily told him who I had met and that she'd been driving forty minutes to my house as often as she could. He asked, "Why isn't she your girlfriend? I don't think she's driving here for her health!"

I gave what he said some thought. Did I really like her? When I first met her, I wasn't that much into her; she was cute, but nothing special. As time passed, from talking to her and seeing her, my emotions increased daily. I enjoyed talking, cuddling and being with her. But was I ready to make it official and open Pandora's box? Had I been struck by the "Love Bug"? I thought, *Maybe. So I'll make her my girlfriend and see what happens.*

We saw each other frequently, going out to eat, the movies, a baseball game, and the beach that summer. And of course, communicated twenty-four/seven. I felt it was a great summer and that nothing could go wrong.

## "Summer's Over" Sorrow

When I went back to college I was happy that I had a girlfriend and was thinking it was going to be a great school year. Unfortunately, all good things come to an end. The first day I got back to college, Rochelle called me crying. She didn't know what to do. She had an eight credits nursing class that had a test every week. She was telling me she didn't know how she was going to do it and didn't feel that she would have time for me. Also, she felt less happy the last two weeks of the summer, maybe because there were times I was insensitive towards her. I promised we would go to the beach by the end of the summer. Her uncle had a medical problem and I hadn't handled the situation the best way because I convinced her to come to the beach instead of seeing her uncle. As you grow older, you learn how to handle situations better. Sometimes it takes more than once, and longer than you'd like, to learn from your mistakes. I pleaded with her not to end the relationship, but she ultimately felt I deserved someone better than her, even after I tried everything to change her mind.

What had happened was not the way I felt our relationship would have ended. When I first started seeing Rochelle, some of my friends told me that she was a little big and that I could do better than her. I kept thinking about their feedback, so I didn't appreciate the relationship as much as I should have when we were together. If you really like someone, don't listen to others' opinions. Just focus on your relationship.

Unfortunately, when someone goes through sadness and is in a slump, people react to it differently. I wasn't one of those people who handled the change in a positive way. To say the least, it was a rough few months. There were times I was so sad that I behaved out of my norm. Specifically, I was speaking in a very forward way towards new girls I was interested in.

75

If you have trauma to the brain, this can change your behavior. I've heard stories from doctors that they have had patients, male and female, who were forward and sexual with others. We need to understand that it can take time to establish a filter. I believe that when someone damages certain parts of their brain, it changes their behavior. I hurt the part that affected my inhibitions and memory, so that could have had some impact on my filter. With frontal lobe injuries, a person with a traumatic brain injury doesn't always know how to behave appropriately.

I have a friend whose sister had an injury similar to mine and she behaved just like me when relationships ended that had involved codependency, which is being dependent on other people. When such a relationship ends, the person who is dependent goes through different types of depression. It's harder for a person with a serious brain injury to let go of emotions. For me personally, it was easier to get over my car accident and just focus on getting better. Why? Because there was nothing I could have done to change the result from my accident. But with my relationship, I would always wonder: If I had done things differently, would we still be together? So coping with the emotions of a breakup was more difficult. Once we figure out how to handle those emotions, life moves more smoothly and we can laugh at how silly we were. I know everybody goes through breakups; I am not alone in this. But research has shown it is a little more difficult after a TBI.

## Dreadful Start to a New Semester

After the breakup, I dwelled on the negatives, rather than embrace the positives of my experience with Rochelle, who was having a tough, long nursing class and getting some experience in the hospital. This at least motivated me to be occupied as well.

As a result, I applied for an internship. This way, I spent my time doing something productive towards my career.

I received an email that fall that a new business had opened in Wilkes-Barre, the city where my college is located, and they were looking for an intern. This business delivered food from numerous restaurants in that region through online orders. I was lucky enough to be granted an opportunity to help them start this new, exciting business. Since I didn't have quite enough college credits needed, sixty, to make this experience an internship for credits, I was considered a volunteer/intern. This was a good experience. I was part of a team that was starting a new business. I helped in strategizing, advertising in person, and using social media to bring awareness to them.

With this sudden end to a relationship, I still wasn't enthusiastic, and my personality with my peers was subdued. Unfortunately, this negatively affected my schoolwork concentration. One class I was excited to take was acting for non-theater majors. The previous semester I'd been gutsy enough to join the lip-syncing contest and do something I wouldn't have done in the past. This new acting class was going to be great, being able to joke around and have fun with it. Unfortunately, the three traits I needed to have in order for me to do well in this class—enthusiasm, being outgoing, and being able to show emotions—were now gone.

The first day, which was the night after Rochelle's breakup with me, the teacher asked the students if they were excited to be back at King's and how we were doing. Everyone who answered responded in a positive and uplifting way to please the teacher. I couldn't muster the attitude to say something positive or enthusiastic so I ignored her first question and said, "Uh, okay." She responded, "Just okay?" And I responded with a quick, aggravated voice, "Yeah." For the first month or two, I didn't care to be enthusiastic while participating in this acting class. Too much sadness and regret were in my mind. It got to the point where, when my midterm grades came out, I had a *B–*.

When I saw my grade, I was aggravated! I knew I could do better if I put effort into it, but my teacher didn't know that. The next class I told her, "I am going to improve a lot. The reason I wasn't that good was because my girlfriend had broken up with me the first day back to school." She told me, "That's why this class is great. You're able to put everything behind you for an hour and just have fun." I took that approach for the class.

A few weeks later we had to pick a song and lip-sync it to the class. This was going to be good. Even though I was nervous in the competition, I'd enjoyed the experience. This time I had more time to ponder which song would be the best to lip-sync. I couldn't decide what song to choose. At first I was thinking of doing a song from an unknown artist. But Tyrone was urging me not to pick a "mix-tape" song, so I chose a popular song, "The Show Goes On," by Lupe Fiasco. I'd listened to that song a lot that summer. Perfect!

This time I decided to prepare more. I went on YouTube and watched Lupe Fiasco sing this song in concerts. This way I wouldn't be stuck doing the same exact movements over ten times, like I had in the contest with the song "Build Me Up, Buttercup" when I pointed up and down and walked around to point at the audience. I had a plan this time; I had more time to prepare. In some of his concerts he wore sunglasses and would raise them up for a few seconds when the lyrics, "Tell them look at me, boy," came on. I was going to do the same thing. I also knew what to do with my hands this time.

The day of the lip-syncing exercise arrived. I was slightly nervous, but more excited to lip-sync this song. I had practiced many times and had a plan. After the first two students did their song, she called my name and was ready to play my song. I approached the small stage, wearing clothes similar to what Lupe Fiasco would wear. As my song began, I felt confident, wearing a plaid button-down shirt that hung over my dark blue jeans and wearing sunglasses that allowed me to hide my eyes and any slight intimidation. As the song played, I paced around, and I knew when to point my fingers and use my hands. Once it hit the time to reveal my eyes for a few seconds, I became even more confident for the remaining minute and a half of the song. After I showed my eyes, I felt as if I wanted the song to last longer.

The teacher thought I did a good job, but that it was a hard song to do with the lyrics moving quickly. I was happy with how I'd done, but I understood where she was coming from. After class, a girl told me that she was surprised I didn't do "Build Me Up, Buttercup" again, since I'd already preformed with that song before. Shocked, I said, "Oh, you saw me in the lip-syncing contest?" She ended up telling me that she was in the first row. After I did the class-assigned lip-syncing exercise, I retired from the college's lip-syncing contests because there wasn't a thrill anymore. I was tempted, but was never excited enough to go through with it.

I had to get through some tough classes in my business courses that semester. One was accounting, the course I had to retake from the first semester. This was something I absolutely did not look forward to. The next was microeconomics, which surprised me. I had just taken macroeconomics at a community college in the summer. *Macro has to be more difficult than micro, right?* I thought. *I should have a general idea about this economic course.* Well, another one of those incorrect assumptions again.

Macroeconomics is a broader concept of economics, where micro is more about being a business owner. That made this class, in my opinion, actually more difficult. It didn't help that the professor didn't speak English well. This confused everyone in the class. It was already a tough class, but made even worse when we could barely understand what the teacher was teaching! I ended up getting a tutor, someone who, when he spoke, I could understand.

None of my classmates were good at this class, so practically everyone failed their tests. This let the teacher curve our grades, and I ended with a respectable grade. Even though I passed the class and have a fair understanding about microeconomics, I enjoyed and understand macroeconomics much more. Education is partially based on the teacher.

Accounting. No more forgetting about it; I had to pass this course for my marketing major. Since I knew it was going to be challenging, I got a tutor immediately. This time I chose my tutor and knew she was going to be really helpful; she was the same girl who had helped me with my finite math class the previous semester. My accounting teacher went fairly quickly through chapters so we could have more time to do practice accounting problems. It took time, but I got used to her teaching style, with outside help from a great tutor. The next semester I had to take the second accounting class. I was lucky enough to have the same teacher and tutor. It was still a difficult course, but knowing my teacher and tutor and their styles of teaching and reviewing, I was finally able to understand it.

## An Effort for a Happier Semester

A path to being happier and clear-minded was important. I had begun to get over Rochelle as the fall semester drew to a close. But two weeks before the semester's end, I faced a situation. I knew a girl that I saw in the game room several times.

This girl could sense when interacting that I thought she was cute. She dated a friend of mine for about a week, but something happened and they broke up. The day after the breakup, she messaged me on Facebook and asked if I wanted to get together. The plan was for her to sleep over. I felt that I had gotten over Rochelle enough and that it would be okay. I hadn't kissed a girl in a few months, and it was almost as if I needed something. But first I had to ask the friend who had dated her if it was okay. He said, "I don't care. She's crazy!"

I decided, *Okay, she can sleep over.* But when I lay on the bed with her, all I could think about was Rochelle. I felt that Rochelle was more attractive than this girl, and that made it worse. Plus, clearly I wasn't ready to move on yet. Unfortunately, this led me into a path of restarting my emotions of getting over someone. The worst thing was that I missed Rochelle even more than I did when she broke up with me.

In order to get over Rochelle, I felt it would be best to not go to parties and talk to girls. There were even times over this breakup when I was thinking of giving a speech about brain injuries, so I could see her again at the city hospitals. A week or so later I was motivated to do it for *me, patients* and *families* I would be speaking to, not to just be near her! That was a confusing and depressing time. Now I can only shake my head and laugh at that emotional thought process of wanting to be around her and at the same time wanting to get over the breakup. I guess I just wasn't ready for a relationship at that time.

On the bright side, I always said I was going to write a book, even when I was a patient in A.I. duPont Hospital! Now I had a personal incentive to start writing outlines about everything that happened in my recovery! I guess you've heard of people writing songs after a breakup; well, I started writing my book. I didn't want to end up starting to write notes too late. If I did, the details of the stories might have faded away.

The next challenge I faced involved making a decision. Originally it was decided that I would get an apartment with Tyrone, Anthony, and Fred. My college had a strategy that allowed students to get an apartment through credentials on how many credits you earned. They had a "lottery," and whoever got picked was allowed to choose what apartment or dorm they would like to live. The more credits someone had, the more lottery picks they received.

Since my friends and I were only sophomores, we didn't have a great chance to win the lottery for our junior year. Fortunately, I found that I had an option of being exempt from the lottery, having had a traumatic brain injury. Luckily, an ADA disability apartment was available in the exact apartment where I wanted to live. This was going to be great! No stress about trying to get into an apartment. I would be close and not have to walk far to classes; I could sleep in a spacious room and spacious apartment, making it easier to live.

However, this apartment only roomed three people, not four, so I had to choose which friend would be eliminated from the apartment. After lots of thinking and discussion with them, the decision was made to not room with Fred. He understood the situation and that we didn't have a great chance of winning the lottery, so he was fine with it.

Academically, I had a rocky start with a few of my classes. Once again, I had underestimated how much I needed to prepare for tests. Also, I knew how much of a workload accounting was going to require in order to pass, so I devoted a lot of time to accounting. I managed to bring my grades up to a good mark and was able to get involved with the business club.

# Chapter Nine
## *Intern Summer*

*There is no exercise better for the heart than*
*reaching down and lifting someone up.*
*—John Holmes*

This summer I completed two experiences that would help prepare me for my future endeavors. These two things were an internship at the nearby hospital marketing and public relations department, and a public speaking event about brain injuries at the Ronald McDonald House, where I had once stayed. All of this was good. I was active in trying to help my career and keep busy.

I had learned a lesson: not to see someone unless you were truly ready. This was because that could make everything even worse than you could imagine. I still wanted nothing to do with women!

With the internship at the hospital, I was lucky that my mom worked there and had connections, which gave me a better chance to get the internship. Also, it helped that, in the beginning, I was the only one who was interning there, so there was no competition.

This internship was a good experience. After my car accident, I became interested in a career in the business aspect of healthcare. Getting the experience in working for a nonprofit organization was good. It allowed me to see how nonprofits operate. Basically, nonprofits get more benefits from the government. These benefits are needed to help the community.

Working nine to five on days that I didn't have a summer class kept me busy, and I saw firsthand what it would be like to work with marketing and public relations in the future. Editing and writing papers about the hospital for newspapers, using Excel for data on a list of people, conducting research about their hospital, its competitors, advertising, etc.—it was a good start for me.

## Preparation

When the summer of my junior year began, my dad contacted the social worker at the Ronald McDonald House and asked if I could give a speech to the patients and parents about brain injuries. She was delighted and granted permission. Before I was to give the speech later that summer I needed to write an outline of what I was going to say. When writing a speech, it's always good to get a second opinion about what to discuss and how to phrase it.

I remembered that Rochelle learned about traumatic brain injuries that previous semester. When I was with her, I was secretly excited about that. But now she's history! I'll be excited in a different way: I'll secretly use her. I may have actually had a slight interest and curiosity to talk to her again, but I had to put that aside. I would never completely get over her if I thought that way. What I really wanted was information, the education she had just learned! I wanted her to feed me ideas on what to include for my first speech on brain trauma, without her being aware she was helping me.

As soon as my great volunteer opportunity was official, I messaged Rochelle on Facebook. I typed in a friendly manner and asked how she had been, how nursing was. This led me to what I actually wanted to hear, without telling her about my public speaking opportunity and my true intentions in talking to her. We gradually started to discuss what she had learned that semester. The information she told me wasn't really descriptive. She told me, "I didn't learn much." Since I couldn't get any details out of her, she was almost useless to me now. After that, I removed her from my friends list. This was something I should have done a long time ago; I had been hurting myself, having the ability to see her face on my chat sidebar. *Now,* I thought, *I'll completely erase you from my memory and move on!*

When I began to write the outline, I had so much bottled up in my mind on what I wanted to say, but I didn't know how I wanted it to be structured. Since this information was going to be 100% based on my experience and not any information from others, I made a tree of information of what I wanted to discuss. For example, with motivating through the recovery, I had one main detail in the middle, with pieces of information connected through lines surrounding that one piece. This strategy was good. It allowed me to connect the information that I wanted to say and in which order to say it.

After seeing the tree of ideas, I wrote my ten-minute speech quickly during the next couple of hours. I had my dad review it, and I reviewed it numerous times to see if anything needed to be changed. Once I wrote the final version of my speech, I practiced it *many times*. I felt it was important to master how I wanted to articulate my words in different parts of the speech, pace myself so that it would be ten minutes, and to know it by heart. I even recorded myself four different times, reading the speech. Whenever I recorded the speech, I put it on my iPod and listened to myself speak; that way, I could hear how I wanted to sound and remember the order in which I would tell my experiences in recovery.

## Showtime—Part 1

No turning back. The day to give my speech had come. I listened to my speech a few times in the car ride to the Ronald McDonald House, trying to know exactly what I was going to say. In the car I was a little nervous, but I was confident that I was prepared enough and that I could give the speech with my eyes closed.

My family and I walked into the Ronald McDonald House. I felt calm and ready to give the speech. First the social worker had to give the weekly updates and rules and information to the families who resided at the house, so I was standing off to the side behind a partition. She finished talking about all of the information that she needed to remind the families about, and then she called my name and introduced me to the audience.

As I stepped to the lectern, I placed my outline on top of it, in case I needed to refer to it. *Immediately*, my legs started to shake and my heart was beating heavily! I had prepared religiously for this speech, and it was about something close to my heart, so it should have been easy. *Right!* Well, the practice helped. Before I gave my speech, I told them my name and said that this was the first time I was speaking to an audience on this subject; I was hoping my nervousness would go away.

Immediately I noticed this one teenager, who I was told later happened to have suffered a traumatic brain injury from an off-road motorcycle racing accident. The entire time I gave the speech, he had his eyes wide open at me, with hope and focus. This didn't ease my nerves one bit; throughout my speech, I kept looking at him and tried to glance at the entire audience.

My speech started off with a fast pace. I was glancing at my speech outline every time I started the next bullet point, as a reminder of what story I was going to tell. This went on for the first few minutes. At the beginning of my speech I spoke about my injury and going through therapies. Once I was about a third of the way into my speech about going to college, I started to calm down. This led me to speak more slowly and soak in the experience. Gaining confidence is *huge* when giving a speech! Once I developed this confidence, I began to speak in a more forceful tone during the parts I was trying to emphasize.

When I finished the speech, a few parents, and the wide-eyed patient came up to congratulate me. This patient said that I gave him inspiration and more motivation to go through his therapies. I was pleased to hear the appreciation of my recovery and that my speech was powerful for them. Even though I was aggravated at myself about how I spoke in the beginning of my speech, this gave me more reassurance, motivating me to continue to write outlines of my experiences in recovery to guide me when writing a more detailed account so that in the future this book would be written. I did not want to put myself in the mindset of "I will someday write this book," possibly leading me into never writing the memoir. If there was at least one more person or family who could get inspiration from my experience, then it would be worth it. Hope, which is a Divine gift, can change attitudes and be a great motivator.

# Showtime—Part 2

While I was preparing for that speech at the Ronald McDonald House, I got a phone call from Mrs. Smith, the Academic Skills program coordinator at King's College. She presented me with an interesting public speaking opportunity. After the first few weeks of the new semester, a Pennsylvania State Representative was going to make a presentation for faculty members about college sport-related concussions and brain injuries and about going to college classes. Even though their presentation was about brain injuries from college sports and going to classes, I was still relevant enough to partner with them and do the presentation for the faculty members. My injury hadn't happened from a college athletic event, and my injury was more than likely much more severe than those college athletes who were injured.

But I did have a brain injury and could give valuable information about some struggles going to classes after this brain trauma. My dad also gave a short speech, from the parent's point of view, of my experience in the hospital. This allowed me not to have to speak about myself in the hospital, where I knew less detailed information. He experienced it and could give his perspectives and account of that timeframe.

I had now gained the experience of giving a speech about myself with a brain injury, which gave me confidence before I did this second speech. For this speech, though, I took a different approach. The second speech was similar to the one I had given a month prior. I'd practiced it many times and it was fresh in my mind. I added some new information about education and took parts out of my first speech to create this next one. Since I was back in classes, I felt comfortable enough with my material not to need to practice as much as before.

My family had driven to my college so they could watch and participate in the presentation. We went right to the building where the presentation was to be held. I was not as nervous this time, so my nerves did not affect my emotions for this speaking engagement. This was a completely different feeling, compared to my first speech. As I listened to my dad speak about my injury, I silently told myself, *Just relax and speak slowly.*

Now it was my turn to speak. I walked up to the stage. I would drink from a water bottle, making sure I was hydrated enough. As I introduced myself and began to tell my story, I remained relaxed, focusing on not speaking too fast, since I was angry with myself about that in the first speech. With this speech, I articulated well the entire time.

This speech gave me a different feeling of satisfaction. Giving the speech to a different type of audience—one that wasn't currently facing those difficult life struggles—let me feel less excitement. Don't get me wrong; I enjoy speaking about brain trauma to a purposeful audience. But this was a more informative type of speech, along with having an inspirational and motivational message within it. Different audiences take away different things from an informational/motivational type of speech. But the one thing I saw that is always there is a sense of hope, and that miracles from Above can and do happen.

I was glad that I expanded my platform of speaking engagements and could now give different types of speeches about brain trauma.

# Chapter Ten
## *Twenty-One*

*When you're young you're not afraid of*
*what comes next.*
*You're excited by it.*
*—Dave Grohl*

In the first few weeks of my junior year of college I turned twenty-one. This allowed me to legally purchase and drink alcohol. Because I sustained a severe traumatic brain injury, doctors didn't recommend drinking alcohol. At least that was the case when I was underage and in the first few years of my recovery. Realistically speaking, the doctors said we all know that students underage at college go to parties and drink. First they advised me that it was illegal and also advised me not to drink; but if I did, not to have more than four ounces of beer. With my injury being a few months less than four years, doctors were more lenient on my consuming alcohol, though they still advised against it.

The deal was four to eight ounces of alcohol that is five percent or lower ABV, alcohol by volume. If you have had a brain injury, the amount and severity of alcohol might be different for you, so talk to your doctor about that. I talked to Dr. Sugarman about it, and he told me I could have one bottle or can of beer. No one is going to drink just four ounces or have just half a beer. My dad always said I was negotiating for a full can of beer instead of sticking to four ounces.

When you're in college, finally being twenty-one can be a big thing. You finally have the power to purchase and drink alcohol and not be reliant on other people to get it for you. And you are able to go out to bars rather than house parties. As time passes, once you've turned twenty-one, alcohol isn't as big a deal, since it can be on hand in your refrigerator. And when the RA in your college dorm checks your room or apartment, having alcohol becomes no worry.

For me, I was excited to turn twenty-one so I could finally go to bars. I wasn't a big fan of house parties, which were run by a frat house or a group of sports players. When I was under twenty-one, I walked around the city, mostly with Tyrone. I saw three types of bars; standard bars, sports bars, and club bars. They looked awesome and I would finally be of age to get the "bar experience." Being a huge sports fan, I was looking forward to being able to sit at the bar, drink a beer and watch a sports game. The club scene looked cool, but I wasn't a good dancer and my legs got tired, so that probably wasn't going to be my first choice of where I'd drink.

The night I turned twenty-one, I had a friend, a grade above me, who wanted to bring me to a bar. I was excited. I've seen Dos Equis commercials and I felt they were cool, being "The most interesting man in the world," so I wanted that to be my first legal drink.

My friend told me which bar to meet him at and what time. As I walked to the bar I was excited and nervous at the same time. The only time I'd sat at a bar was when I went to New York

City for a college-funded advertising trip, where I drank water and watched the Phillies in a playoff game. I hoped I'd be able to sit down at the bar, chill and watch sports. As I approached the bar, the windows were dark and I was unable to judge what kind of scene that I'd be going into. As I walked in I saw lots of adults dancing. That was kind of intimidating. Many of these people were older than me. This left me kind of shocked and uncomfortable. I saw my friend and another person, so I walked up and greeted them. They welcomed me in and showed me all the parts of the bar and bought me a drink. Being with people I knew gave me some sense of comfort, embracing the partying with people older than me.

I walk with my two friends through the crowd of people. As I continue to walk with them, I saw someone I knew. It was Rochelle. *Are you kidding me?* I was trying to write her out of my life and now I saw her, out of all the people, and I had only been there ten minutes! Seeing her and her friends made me feel even more uncomfortable. It was new enough trying to absorb the new adult scene, but now I was thinking of her again.

I told my friend that I had seen Rochelle with her friends. He said, "That's cool. I'll say hi to them." How I met Rochelle was actually through my friend, who I was with at the bar for the first time when we went to the eighteen-and-over dancing club. He went over to them without me to say hi. I hadn't seen her in a year, but now, whenever I'd go out, there was a good chance I'd see her again. Lovely! It hurt my first bar experience. Later I thought it would be best if I happened to see her in the future not to let it hurt my experience. Instead, be respectful and wave hello or something like that, rather than look the other way and let it get in my head.

## Before I Ran Towards My Goals

As I mentioned earlier, with my plan of getting over Rochelle, I felt it was important to isolate myself from girls until I was ready. After that long break of focusing on myself, I felt maybe I was ready. When the new school year began, I felt more confidence about communicating with girls again. This led me to do some casual dating. Unfortunately, none of those dates led to anything serious.

For one of my classes I had to do a presentation. I had completed my presentation at night, so I could practice my presentation. But there was a problem: The printer in my room had run out of ink. The easiest way for me to print my presentation was to go to my apartment computer lab. When I walked into the small computer lab, there was only one computer available. I walked to the available computer to print my file. Sitting next to me was a nice, outgoing, and attractive girl. I had felt I was ready to talk to girls again, so this was a great opportunity. We talked for a few minutes and I thought she was pretty cool. I wondered if I'd ever see her again, since I hadn't been alert enough to ask for her number or add her on Facebook.

The following month after I met the girl at the computer lab I was with a friend and his large group of friends. We decided to go to a bar for a drink and to meet some girls. When I went to a bar, I had always been cautious to make sure I drank only the one beer. I really wanted to feel loosened up from a beer and dance with girls that night.

You'll remember that I had weak legs and poor balance after I met Rochelle sober at a club, and I could barely stand and walk after two hours. When drinking alcohol, that would make anyone's balance even worse!

So here we were at the bar, a group of guys who wanted to have a good time and dance with girls. Like before, I stood and moved around a lot and my legs become very fatigued. It got to the point where they felt like Jell-O, just like they did the other time. Have you ever had the feeling that your upper body weighs a hundred pounds and your legs can only carry ten pounds? When that happens, it just doesn't look good when you walk or stand.

It had gotten so bad that a few times I had to lean against a pool table no one was playing on, to help me stand up. While leaning against the pool table, I started to lose balance and my back fell onto the pool table. I ended up lying on the table for at least fifteen seconds, so I put my arms back to rest. A guy finally took notice and said, "Hey, man, I don't think you're allowed to do that."

Laughing, I responded, "I can't get up." So to get me off the pool table, he pulled me up.

I really needed to rest my legs and relax. I knew there was a bench outside, so that's where I was headed; it was too difficult for me to sit on those high stools in the bar. I needed to get outside. My legs were extremely fatigued, and my balance was getting worse. Nothing was going to stop me. I mean nothing!

When I got off the pool table I saw the exit, and that's where I wanted and needed to be. It was crowded in the bar that night, and a big group was blocking the exit. The only way to get to the exit was to walk there. I said "Excuse me" as I bumped into people as lightly as possible. Towards the end of the walk to the exit I saw one of Rochelle's friends and gave her an even harder bump than the rest of the crowd. Finally, I reached the exit!

Once I got outside, my body started to lean back at a forty-degree angle. Surprisingly, I was able to walk. I thought, *Wow, I never experienced this before. How am I still standing and walking?* Then I looked to my right and saw Rochelle standing outside, talking to a guy. But I ignored them. I had my eyes locked on the open bench.

I reached the bench and sat down for a few minutes and relaxed. The guy Rochelle was talking to came up to me and said, "Hey, I'm Rochelle's friend. She asked me to come over and see if you're okay." I told him that I was fine and said thanks.

I guess it's not every day that you see someone you know walking in such a ridiculous manner. My body was so slanted back that I looked extremely intoxicated, even though I wasn't actually drunk.

After ten minutes, I was confident that my legs were rested enough to stand, so I walked back into the bar. As I went back inside, a girl came up to me, asking, "Are you okay?" I responded, "Yeah, I'm fine." She said, "Do you remember me?" I thought, *Not really*, and told her that I didn't. She told me she was Vicky and that we met at the computer lab last month. I said, "Oh, okay! Yeah, I know you. Do you want to dance?" She said, "Um, I don't think you can stand up enough to dance." I tried to show her that my legs were rested enough to dance. Eventually, though, I agreed that it was probably best not to dance.

## Running Towards My Goals

After that night I got to know Vicky better. A week or two later, we went to a pizza shop and she told me that a girl had come up to her right after she got done speaking to me at the bar that infamous night. That girl was Rochelle. Rochelle had told her in a defensive manner, "Hey! You know that's my ex-boyfriend!" Rochelle was intoxicated, so it's hard to know exactly how she felt. Vicky had interpreted the confrontation to be jealousy. At the time I was pleased to hear that news, thinking maybe Rochelle still cared for me and I'd made her jealous. But I had to tell myself it didn't matter, because she was history, and I tried not to dwell on the past.

As I got to know Vicky better, I became interested in getting together with her more often. She wanted to go to grad school to study physical therapy. She became interested in becoming a physical therapist when her cousin had a brain tumor and had to go through therapies similar to what I'd had to go through. She was already very athletic and really good at track, so it was fitting for her.

Winter break came a month later, and I had a sudden desire to be able to run again. My walk and coordination had improved tremendously. I decided to call up the athletic desire that I once had with swimming, to be able to run. This would improve my coordination and allow me to be closer to where I was physically, prior to the car accident.

Years prior, I had tried a few times to run, but I didn't stay motivated like I should have. Schoolwork and my college social life got in the way. Plus, I was content with how I walked. During that break I went to the gym that my mom worked at and focused on my ability to run. My coordination and technique were off. I knew I needed help if I wanted to be able to run well.

When I returned to college, I knew who to talk to about improving my running ability. I talked to Vicky, the girl who wanted to become a physical therapist and was a good track athlete. When I told her what my goal was, she was interested in helping.

I showed her some of the videos of my attempts to run in the past, and it was clear there were some things I needed to work on. We made regular visits to the indoor track at the college to work on my coordination and running ability. She showed me some walking exercises that would better my rhythm while running. We met twice a week, and I began to improve rapidly.

Since she was an athlete and I had been an athlete and was competitive, my determination to run was very focused and intense. Sometimes that approach could be really good. Unfortunately, for me it didn't turn out well. When going through physical therapy-type exercises, moderation throughout the exercises and guidance on what to do by a professional is always the best approach to take.

About a month and a half after doing intense exercises, I started to feel something weird with my right ankle. Whenever I ran, I started to feel this agonizing pain there. It was weird, though. When I was walking I felt no pain. But whenever I ran, the pain would start. I wanted to reach my goal of running and spend time with Vicky, so I ignored the problem with my right ankle.

At first I could run for fifteen minutes, and then I would start to feel the pain in my right ankle. Then it gradually got worse and I felt it after five seconds. She was concerned and was weary of continuing to help me train. It was difficult to explain. How could my ankle be one hundred percent fine when walking, but painful when I ran?

I was stubborn, not wanting to let anything get in the way of my being able to run. Tyrone was a person I felt confident talking to about injuries, since he played football in high school, lifted daily, and knew a lot about muscle groups, so I demonstrated for him and pointed to where the pain was. He thought I'd hurt my Achilles tendon. He told me to ease up on the training with Vicky and to not run for now. If I hurt it more, I wouldn't be able to walk!

To get another opinion, I went to the nurse at my college to get my right ankle checked out. The first thing she noticed was that my sneakers were really worn out. She advised me to get newer sneakers and to not strain my ankle anymore, and she taped up my ankle. But I still wanted to be able to run; and how was I to know when my ankle was fixed?

Tyrone and I felt my ankle might be better if it was taped. I went to the track with him once or twice to see how it felt. After running with him, I was delighted to see that my ankle didn't hurt when it was taped. I wised up, not wanting to hurt myself, and delayed my training until I saw a physical therapist about my injury.

## Physical Therapy

A month later my semester ended. I thought I'd hurt my Achilles tendon when training, but I wasn't a doctor, so I wanted to see a physical therapist. That injury can be serious business. If I really hurt it, it would keep me from walking, so it was decided I should go back to my old physical therapy place, Achieve, just to get it checked out.

I explained this odd injury to George, my old physical therapist; that I could walk with no pain, but if I ran I'd then feel agonizing pain. He felt my ankle and checked it out by having me do different exercises to see what it could be. The result became clear: I had hurt my tibialis posterior.

What's a tibialis posterior? It's a key stabilizing muscle in the lower leg, located on the top of the foot, next to the ankle. But how did I get this injury? Whenever I ran, my foot positioned outward. After the extensive training, I put too much pressure on the outside of my foot and ankle, and that's what led to the injury. This explained the mystery, why my ankle would hurt when running and not walking. While walking I wasn't putting as much pressure on my foot.

To correct this injury, I went to physical therapy for about a month. Something that was important to help fix the injury was to walk with my right foot going straight, rather than pointing outward. There had been volleyball athletes in the Olympics who hurt their shoulders while playing. The solution was to put elastic therapeutic tape on the injured shoulder to help the athletes play to their best ability without any pain.

My therapist wanted to be creative with helping my injury and allowing me to run again, so he did some experiments, taping elastic therapeutic tape around my calf, foot, and ankle. After a few tries, he figured out where the tape had to be placed to protect the injury from recurring. The goal of the tape was to correctively force me to point my toes straight. This would allow me to run, putting equal pressure on my foot and ankle, all while not damaging the tibialis posterior. After walking, running, and doing many exercises to loosen and strengthen my ankle, it healed enough to the point where physical therapy was no longer needed for that injury.

## Thanks?

Before that semester ended, I knew it might be the last time I saw some of the seniors. That meant it was possible I'd never see Rochelle again. I thought I was pretty close to one hundred percent over her, but something irritated me. She didn't know that she had sparked interest in me to do speaking engagements about brain trauma, how I started to keep a journal for a book in the future, and that she had unknowingly affected my life. I felt it was right for her to know. Occasionally, these thoughts would slip into my mind when I tried to sleep. Something needed to be done.

Even though I wasn't friends with her on Facebook, I was still able to message her, so that's what I did. I expressed to her that I might not see her again and there was something I'd like to tell her about how she helped me recover from my traumatic brain injury and unknowingly introduced new possibilities for me and gave me a push to start something. I indicated I would rather see her in person to explain it, though.

She didn't respond! Well, I tried. She didn't want to hear it, so there was no reason to feel bad anymore. I told my roommate Tyrone about it, and he was angry. He already hated her, after seeing how I was so sensitive after her breaking up with me. He said, "If you did see her, what would you tell her, that her acting like a bitch changed your life? She doesn't deserve shit, dude! Also, she probably thinks you want to get with her. Forget her!"

My close friend Willis, from back home, strongly disliked Rochelle as well. He hadn't even been fond of her when I was dating her. He was one of the friends who gave me grief for being with her in the first place, feeding into my brain that I deserved better than her. He said, "Let me remind you, the girlfriend you had when you were in high school was pretty and thin; how can you go from that to this?" I told him it didn't matter; I was attracted to her physically and mentally. He was just trying to be a friend who looked out for me.

When the breakup happened, I had vented to Willis about my sadness and regret on how I'd acted and gave some blame towards him for not encouraging me during the relationship and instead criticizing it. He got sick of seeing her name through my texts! After the breakup, he kept telling me, "She deserves no credit with the idea of starting your book and speaking engagements. You said yourself that when you were messed up in the hospital you thought of writing a book. She deserves nothing!" After that I understood where he was coming from, and that what he'd said was true.

He was adamant that she shouldn't even be mentioned in the book. But I told him, "What happened is important for anyone to read, especially a person who has had a brain injury. It is perfect for this book! It may be difficult for a reader to cope with changes." If Willis ever found out that I'd messaged Rochelle with the hope of getting together to express how my life changed, along with beginning to write notes and speak about brain trauma, I don't know how he'd react. More than likely, he would send me a text that simply said, "SMH." This meant "Shake my head." That was his trademark saying to me. Well, she blew it; that's all I wanted to say. If she wants to find out, she can buy the book.

# Chapter Eleven
## *Luck Be a Lady*

*A gambler is nothing but a man who*
*makes his living out of hope.*
*—William Bolitho*

Before I turned twenty-one I always had some interest in going to a casino. With my brain injury, I couldn't get "hammered," or should I say drunk, like other people, so that took away some excitement. But at the casino I wasn't limited on how much I could gamble. The problem was, the casino was far enough away from the college that you would have to drive there.

My roommate Anthony had turned twenty-one months after I did. He definitely had an interest in gambling and going to a casino. Later on, he ended up working in a casino, counting money in the early mornings.

The first time I went to a casino, Anthony had me do slots in the beginning. I got bored, just pushing a button, watching numbers or pictures circle around and hope that they landed your way. After watching him play slots some more, I wanted to do something else. When I was a kid, I had played poker with my friends. If I was to play poker at the casino, I would be there for countless hours. He mentioned that he had liked the game blackjack, which he played when he went to the casino a few weeks prior. We decided to find a cheap buy-in and play blackjack, also known as 21. I saw a movie about blackjack and understood that the goal was to get 21, but I was very new to the game.

I approached the five-dollar buy-in table and saw there was only one seat available, so I decide to join the game. I threw in the five dollars and got one chip. More decks were rolled, and next thing I knew, I had forty dollars. As the hours went by, I continued to play and learn more while I played. Luck was on my side that night. I didn't know the strategies of the game—when to "hit" or "stand"—all I knew was that I wanted to get 21. Since I didn't think logically when the right time was to "hit" or "stand," I got my fair share of losses. But this night turned out to be my first night of luck.

In some hands, my two cards would be as high as 18 or 19, but it wasn't 21, so I said "hit," asking to get another card. Miraculously, when doing that I would get a 2 or 3. When I started to bring in more chips, some older people sitting at the table who weren't winning got frustrated, yelling, "Come on, that's a bust card!" "Why would you hit on that?" "Don't stand on that card!" Or their anger would show through their facial expressions.

Later in the game, I was grateful to have other players guide me on what to do. This probably was also to help them, hoping that the dealer would bust his own hand, going above 21, and all the players would win. I started to really enjoy the game and got a rush of excitement. Hours flew by so fast. It got late, and my ride, Anthony, wanted to leave. I counted my chips with glee, doing it nice and slow. I was at two hundred dollars, and I'd only spent the minimum, five dollars!

## Addictive Tendencies

Anthony and I ended up going to the casino once every other week for two months. The "rush" of playing blackjack became more intense each time I went. That semester, I didn't do as nicely with my winnings, and sometimes I lost money. It was okay; I only brought forty dollars I was willing to gamble. Now that I had two hundred dollars extra to spend, it wasn't that big a concern. I mean, I was only spending "casino money." I didn't have that two hundred dollars before I went to the casino that lucky night. Plus, it was a night out. If you go to an event or a restaurant, you are going to spend money. If you had fun, that's all that mattered. With the casino, I could even earn money! It was strictly entertainment money.

As the weeks passed, I couldn't wait to play blackjack again! I was even excited to smell the pleasant scent of stepping into the casino; it was nice and refreshing. I even told my roommates, Anthony and Tyrone, that I wish there was cologne that had the same scent as the casino; it was that good!

Tyrone wasn't fond of the idea of Anthony and me going to the casino so often. He said that I didn't hide my emotions well. He could instantly tell how I did when I got back to the apartment. If I was happy, I did well; if I was frustrated, I lost money.

Since I wasn't an expert on how to play blackjack, I wanted to be better prepared. That first night was lucky. Risky decisions weren't going to happen all the time. If I knew how to strategize better, I'd win more often! Or so I thought. I downloaded a free blackjack app on my phone that used fake money. I became hooked on the game, playing over 1,500 hands in ten days! I started to get bored with the app and felt that I was ready to succeed with real money.

It was a Wednesday in March. Anthony had a test on Friday, and he wanted to drive to the casino a day earlier than our traditional every-other-week Thursday. He wanted to leave immediately from the cafeteria after dinner. I was a little late getting ready to eat, so I grabbed my wallet and left my room.

After we ate, we left for the casino. I was excited and felt confident about playing blackjack. This was my night! I had prepared so much. I was now ready to know when to hit, stay, double down, and split. I arrived at the available table with a feeling of excitement and a rush of finally being able to gamble with real money, not an app with "fake" money.

We started to play blackjack, and I didn't have a great start. I lost my forty dollars, and it had been less than fifteen minutes! I still had a rush to gamble, but I'd lost my chips. What was I supposed to do the next few hours we were going to be there: *Watch* blackjack?

Usually I didn't bring my debit card, because I didn't want to be in a situation where I had to keep withdrawing money in order to gamble. But that time I had my debit card in my wallet. I withdrew fifty dollars, confident that I would at least break even.

I played some new blackjack games and started to finally win. But then I started to lose. My chips began to fade away again! By the time I had just a few chips to play, Anthony was finished and wanted to drive back to our apartment. I was frustrated with my casino experience that night. When walking back to the car, I tried to get rid of my few one dollar chips in slots on our way to the exit. Almost none of the slots accepted such low-valued chips. I don't even know what I ended up doing with the couple dollars of chips I had left.

I didn't want to see Tyrone and listen to him ask how we did. Anthony and I prepared to say that he broke even and I lost money, but not that much.

I opened the door and Tyrone asked how we did. In a frustrated tone, I said, "I did fine." Tyrone could tell that I lost money, so he started to ask, "How much did you lose?" I didn't want to talk about it, so I slammed my bedroom door in his face and locked it so he wouldn't walk into my room, something he did every day.

I stormed into my room, just angry at myself. I'd lost more money than I ever wanted to spend at a casino. Then I looked at the stash of hidden casino money I had won two months prior, which had begun to fade away. I'd expected that money to become thinner, because when I went to restaurants or stores I was able to pay cash, but not this quickly! I was going to bring that money back up, with more victorious casino nights. Even more depressing and frustrating was that I had used my debit card to spend more than I promised myself I would spend.

The next day I was going to have to face Tyrone, since we lived in the same apartment. I just told him that I lost forty dollars and wanted to end the conversation. He could tell that I was lying and that I had really lost more, so I confessed how much I had actually lost. He was concerned, saying, "You are a gambling addict. I don't think you can handle it with your brain functioning the way it does right now, and you should talk to your parents about this. It has become really bad. You slam your door, yell, and aren't able to cope with talking about your gambling experience. You want to go all the time." He was right. And I don't even think Tyrone knew about my playing free blackjack on my phone all the time the week prior. If I had been able to drive myself to the casino, I might have wanted to go every day.

I called my dad and told him about my gambling problem. He said, "I feared this. I knew it wasn't good that you won so much on your first gambling night. I told your aunt, and she was happy that you did well. But I told her, 'He's going to get addicted and think that he might get the idea that he will be lucky every time he goes.'"

He told me a story about someone who had a similar experience with losing money from horse racing and how some people take it to the extreme, that they even gamble with their mortgage money. He didn't want me to get caught up in gambling and lose more money. After arguing that I wasn't addicted, I decided he was right. Maybe my addictive gambling tendencies were getting the best of me. Go to the casino once or twice a year, not once or twice a month! I decided not to go to the casino the rest of the semester and through the summer. I needed a break.

Back to what Tyrone had said about my brain not being able to handle it. I don't think my brain injury was the reason for my addictive gambling tendencies. That can happen to anyone. Addictive gambling can be extremely dangerous, and I'm glad mine didn't get carried away. I'm not an expert on gambling addictions, but I believe in some negative circumstance this could make you feel depressed, frustrated, and angry. The results could be bankruptcy, homelessness, destroyed relationships with your friends, divorce, and theft. I'm sure the list could go on and on, with how the negative feelings and actions of being a gambling addict can affect you. There are several other common addictions: drugs, alcohol, smoking, shopping, and social media. That list also goes on. I believe having a strong supporting group of friends and family is the easiest way to stop an addiction. But that's once you admit you have a problem. That is when you can allow that supporting group to help you fight through that addiction.

## Brain Cells

When you have trauma to your brain, the hope is that you'll be able to progress and function well over time with whatever issues you have. Having a good memory and having good attention skills are important when learning new information with any kind of study, whether it's an educational course, an exercise in speech therapy, or just living life. Yes, a broad statement: *just living life.*

You could have a job, and in order to successfully complete the tasks assigned to you, having those two skills would be important. Those skills matter even in something as simple as going to buy groceries: being able to remember and be attentive enough to get to the store needed, knowing where to get the groceries and knowing which ones to get. There are plenty of neurological skills that can affect anyone who has had trauma to their brain, but in my opinion, in order to do well in college, having a good memory and good attention skills are the two basic essentials to be able to compensate for any deficits one might have.

It is always good to listen and be attentive when learning new information. After one listens to a lecture, being able to remember it for a test or just for general knowledge or when you enter the workforce is equally important. These two semesters of my junior year, academically I did well, having fewer struggles compared to previous semesters. My brain cells had been healing and were exercised as I constantly learned new information to pass my classes. At that point it had been four years since my car accident.

Going to college and challenging my brain, I believe, was one of the reasons why my recovery had gone so well. In my junior year, I thought I had reached the point where I had mentally recovered enough that I wouldn't be faced with the academic struggles I had faced during my first few years of college. However, my senior year gave me an unfavorable surprise that remind me I needed to spend plenty of effort on my memory and attention skills.

# Chapter Twelve
## *Senior Year Was Supposed to Be Relaxing, Right?*

*There's going to be stress in life, but it's*
*your choice*
*whether to let it affect you or not.*
*—Valerie Bertinelli*

Senior year had finally arrived. I was excited to be in the same apartment, go to bars, and live up the last year of freedom at college. That feeling is common for seniors in college, wanting to leave with a bang. A strategy that some college students have is to finish their difficult courses early so the senior year can be easier. I took an approach of spreading out difficult courses, doing one or two a semester, along with getting classes done in the summer.

That year my first day of classes seemed good, and there was nothing to be concerned about. However, the next day I had two classes in my business course, and the last class of the day was a different story. It isn't a good sign when on the first day the teacher is saying how difficult the class can get, with thirty-three percent of his students failing, and giving an example on how he is not lenient with students. He gave this example: "If it's the spring semester before you graduate, you have a wife and a child, have a job lined up in Europe, along with a house, if you get a fifty-nine percent in my class, sixty percent being a passing grade; I'm still going to fail you." This wasn't news that I wanted to hear at the start of my senior year. Who gives that as an example the first day of class, talking about how people fail your class? My financial management teacher that semester did.

The teacher for my financial management class made me paranoid, and I lost sleep. For many reasons I lost sleep, actually. Not only because of his analogy the first day, telling us a lot of people fail his difficult class, but I didn't have a tutor yet. The grading was multiple-choice for financial equations. The professor would think of common financial equation errors and make those as options for an answer. He gave no extra-credit assignments, and he had a dumb game for taking quizzes: He had dice, and he would pick two numbers before the class started. These numbers were the numbers that would mean a possible pop quiz. Then a student had to choose a number between one and three, where two of the numbers would mean a similar homework question and the other number mean no quiz. Complicated? Yes, I know.

Every time we had homework, I carefully answered every question. The first two quizzes weren't that bad, but the class became more difficult, as the teacher had warned us. As the questions became more challenging, I'd become nervous about a possible quiz. It got to the point where I always talked about financial management to my roommates, which they eventually found annoying. Often, they could even read what was on my mind.

At last! I finally got a tutor to help me with this class. Sadly, I was already mentally screwed; I had failed a handful of quizzes and was behind on the material, so I had to learn more in a short period of time.

A week or two later it was the first test. To prepare for this test, the teacher gave the students a worksheet of questions. I wanted to be prepared, so I did all these questions three times to feel confident I would do well on the test and to make up for the failed quizzes. When the test started I noticed something odd. Most of these questions were not similar to the worksheet at all! The grade was twelve right, out of twenty-five; I failed the test.

At the end of the next class I went to the teacher and told him how seriously I had studied the worksheet questions, only to find they weren't even relevant to the test. Why was that? He told me in a serious manner, "I don't even know what's going to be on the test. I give a worksheet of possible types of questions. My approach is to go on my computer and give my students random questions from the material in the book. Some I didn't teach as much, but you are supposed to read the book on what I didn't teach."

Irritated, I responded, "Why would you give us a worksheet of questions that aren't going to be helpful for the test?"

The teacher said in a joking way, "If we were playing football, the offensive team wouldn't give the defense their playbook." After hearing him say that, I thought, *Does he treat his job as a game, trying to fail his students?* I just walked out.

For my financial management class, I devoted so much of my time studying the daily homework questions for possible quizzes and the test, I didn't study that hard for my other classes and it hurt my other grades. After that teacher gave me a paper with my overall grade showing I was failing, I went to his office, which I did often to make sure I understood the homework questions before class, to discuss whether I should drop the class or not. He told me that it was going to be hard to pass the class as the material became more challenging, which I noticed. If it was hurting my other classes, then it was best to play it safe and withdraw. My tutor tried to convince me not to withdraw from the class. But honestly, it was the first time in two months I truly had peace of mind. One of my roommates was friends with my tutor, and she told him that she went to see my teacher about my withdrawing from the class. The professor told her, "I know. It was good that he withdrew. He was going to fail."

## A Chance to Fix What Was Broken

After my decision to withdraw from financial management, that didn't mean it was an easy road for that semester. Yes, it was a relief that I no longer had to devote an incredible amount of time to one class, but I still had my other classes to pass. With most of them I hadn't done as well in tests as I'd hoped. But now I'd have the ability to bring those grades up. I figured more freedom available to dedicate more time to them ought to be the answer.

What I predicted about my grades going dramatically up with my decision to stop that class came true. For instance, I didn't do as well on my first test for one of my marketing classes; actually many of the students did poorly. It had been one week since my class schedule opened up, so I wanted to prepare better and get a good grade on that test.

The first test had been difficult. The questions were terms and research strategies applied to real business situations. I had to think of a way to study better for that test. Clearly, just reading over terms and strategies repetitively didn't work well. I thought of an idea, but it was going to take some time to organize.

The next class, a week before the test, I spoke to my teacher about how the last test was hard and that I needed to study differently to get a good grade. I said, "I'm going to make up my own practice tests with all of the information we had learned in those chapters and quiz myself every time I review." He said that was a great idea and that he had never heard of a student doing that for his tests. The teacher agreed to look over my "test" and see if he had any suggestions.

I had already talked to the teacher about my plan, so now I actually *had* to do it. After hours of making up my test with all of the information, I was exhausted. It took two days to finish!

Here are a few examples of the practice test questions I made on Terms and Concepts in the marketing research class.

**Types of data: Interval?** Description, order, distances, 1 to 10 scale, colors. Anything on a scale can be called interval. Rate the Redskins' performance this season. Answer: 4–10.

**Types of scales: Semantic scales?**
Sports teams talents?

Heat (hot)---------------------------------- (cold)76ers
Broncos (hot)------------------------------(cold)Jaguars

**Comparative Scale?**
Rate RG3's performance as a football player compared to last year's stats.
Compare RG3's stats this year compared to last year.
Answer: 2

**Type of research: Convenience?** Sample based on using people who are easily accessible.

**Mall intercept** is a convenience sample. Ask fans in baseball games to fill out an All-Star voting paper while watching the game.

Good idea, right? Well, after quizzing myself and reading over my questions, I felt prepared to do well. The day of the test came, and all I thought of was my questions about sports and other examples I had made that interested me.

When the test started, it seemed so simple. I breezed through that test! What is interval data? I thought of the Redskins. What is semantic scale? Oh, that is a rating, like hot and cold. The Heat being a good team and the 76ers being a bad team came to my mind. What is a comparative scale? Instantly thought of RG3 and knew the answer in a second. Which one is mall intercept? Well, when at a baseball game, it's convenient for the fans to choose the league's All Stars.

Next class our grades were in. The teacher wrote on the board the total amount of grades for each letter. He wrote a lot of *C*s and *D*s and only two *A*s. I was nervous! There were quite a few really smart students in my class; my chances of getting a high grade had suddenly shrunk.

I got an *A*! That means I got a top-two grade! If I had kept that finance course instead of withdrawing from it, I would have been one of those lower grades, not a doubt in my mind. Being able to spend more time studying for this marketing research test was a huge factor in achieving my grade.

I studied more and used the same study approach for a few other classes. My grades went up. If you are in a class and have difficulty taking a test, brain injury or not, try something new that will help you remember that information. When you can think of something that you feel is common sense and can relate that to what you are studying, remembering that information becomes incredibly easier.

# Please Join!

Junior year I was the vice-president for a business club, the one I'd gotten involved in during my second year in college. Unfortunately, this wasn't a popular club for students to join. For the first meeting, the club officers and I decided that we needed a strategy to attract students. The idea was to offer free pizza for the new club members and hope that they would be interested in the club.

In an interesting scenario, it was a rainy day and it was difficult for the teacher, who was the club's advisor, to get the pizza. As a result, the students who had showed up were wondering where the promised pizza was, and they became bored with what was said about the club. Throughout the school year, very few students committed to the club, and with the lack of members it became difficult for us to do anything. It was a mess, which I take some blame for. The majority of the year we did nothing, nor did we spend any money. This didn't look good at all! I felt pressured from the college and was frustrated regarding the direction the club was heading. We needed to actually do something! I asked one of my friends, Henry, to join the club and help us raise money for charity. He agreed. This was great; I wouldn't have to do it all by myself, due to a lack of members to help.

Henry and I set up a bowling event for charity. Since students had no interest in joining the club, it would have been asking too much for them to go out of their way to raise money. College students generally don't have a lot of money and are reluctant to spend what they do have. It would be ideal if I could get the students to have a free game or "ten frames" of bowling. This could be used to raise money for charity.

"Three strikes and you're out"; that's how an at-bat for baseball works. It was spring and the beginning of the baseball season. We needed to have a clever idea for businesses to donate money to our cause. We ended up paying in advance with club monies for the joined students to bowl two games. The idea to pitch to donating businesses was this: For the students' first free ten frames, whenever they got a strike, three dollars would go toward charity from each donating business. Anything else would result in no money. This plan worked. We got a few businesses willing to donate, and we were able to use the club money, which we hadn't used all school year, to pay for the students to bowl.

The turnout was good; we got around twenty-five students to bowl. It was the first time I'd bowled in a long time, so it was interesting. My coordination was getting better, but it wasn't great. I stood still, bent my knees, swung my arm and released the ball from my fingers. No fancy footwork for me. We had a good time and raised about $200 for the charity.

## Leadership

The next school year, my senior year, I was president of the business club. This school year I really wanted a better turnout for the club. I felt that I had learned from the past mistakes I had made and experienced. I had the skills to run a charity event mostly by myself; I didn't really need assistance. Isn't that being a leader?

Even though I felt that I was a leader from last school year's accomplishment, I still didn't know how to be an actual "leader." We had a new teacher advising the club. One time before a club meeting, the new advisor made it pretty clear to me and to Henry, the vice-president, things did need to change. She spoke in a blunt and demanding way towards us. This wasn't a welcoming way to communicate.

After the discussion, or should I say "interrogation," Henry and I had a brief discussion about what to do. We had a club meeting in a few minutes and felt almost threatened by her demands. She had good points; for example, that we should delegate more, and we decided to answer some of what she wished. These wishes were to get members more involved in decisions by having four committees. These committees were responsible for covering different sections of the club. They were to get together and set up their own meetings to brainstorm and coordinate their section of business and propose it to me so it could be discussed in a club meeting. After that they would act upon it themselves. *Really!?* Last school year it was difficult enough for us to have people continue to come to meetings. It wasn't like they were getting paid. They already had a busy schedule with schoolwork. Adding these responsibilities might be too much. We had more committed members that year, which was good. We figured we'd set up two committees and see how that worked.

The next few months after that there were some confrontations between the advisor, whom I strongly disliked, and me. I really tried to avoid her. Almost everyone joined a committee, but that didn't work out well the first month. No one proposed ideas to discuss in the club meetings, and they didn't get together. However, the week before our charity event to raise money for different charities, they came up with an idea. When they started to get the hang of the committees, they began to have meetings of their own.

In the beginning of the semester, the club as a whole came up with an idea to sell candy bars to raise money for charity.

Then the committee came up with a new idea, sell hot chocolates. The problem was that candy bars had already been purchased with the club money, to support the original plan. It was a stressful time, having to set up hot water to sell hot chocolates at the last second. But everything worked out and we all did a great job. The candy bars were sold after three days, and most of the hot chocolates were sold that week. It surprised me that we raised more money for that charity event, compared to the previous semester's bowling event. Having more people involved overall was a good thing. We were a more cohesive and organized group.

The next semester we continued to do more. One notable event was educating Hispanic middle-school students about how their ability to be bilingual was great for the workforce and that they should take advantage of it.

My last semester, I took a leadership class and learned the fundamentals of how to be a leader. Eventually, I thanked the club advisor for strongly suggesting changing how the club was being operated. Being a leader isn't just taking power and completing the task. Many different things go into leadership. The goal is to be able to work with and lead others to completing a task. From the leadership education and the club, I am more prepared to take on a roll as a leader, no matter what level of work I am at.

## Relaxing Winter

I had one more semester left of college. Technically it could be more, but I had sixteen more credits to complete in order to earn my Bachelor's degree, and I had to retake financial management then, too. If it weren't for that class, it would have been an easy last semester. Thirteen credits and I felt that I could handle the rest of my classes. Heck, I had an elective left, and I could have taken a writing class and started this book that semester!

My plans were to use my elective and begin writing this book and to use my last marketing elective on an internship for three credits. I was lucky enough to get an internship for the last semester. This internship was with a marketing design company that was within walking distance of my apartment. In addition, it was an internship within my field of study and was a different type of internship than the ones I'd had previously. It was ideal.

The next step was to find out if this internship could count as my last marketing elective. I went to the president of the business school and he told me that this would not count as a marketing elective. If I wanted to get three credits for this internship, I would have to use a regular elective. That was the one elective I had saved for writing this book, so this led to some heavy pondering.

The first semester of my senior year was over. It was winter break and I was faced with a completely different scenario than I'd imagined:

1. I had sixteen credits left, including a class that had previously given me problems.

2. The internship was not going to count for the type of elective that I wished for.

3. The internship relocated a few blocks to the other side of the city, creating an even longer walk.

4. The internship wouldn't be a paying job, and I wasn't sure I wanted to walk up to 20 minutes each day to volunteer.

My thought process about this book was that I didn't want to be stressed out with my classes, especially with the one I imagined I'd devote lots of my time to, so the use of my last regular elective had to be used for something else, unfortunately. That winter the plan was to get my wisdom teeth removed and just get that out of the way. Let it be a relaxing winter, just healing from the dental surgery.

I didn't want to have sixteen credits my last semester, especially with the finance course still to be taken. So a decision was made! Forego the wisdom teeth surgery and worry about that another time. Instead, take a winter class as my last regular elective. Fortunately, I saw an interesting and easy online class at a local community college: music appreciation. That seemed like it would be fairly simple, just learning about music.

With this online music class being normally five months, they had to compress it: The teacher had a lot to teach in a short amount of time. It was more time consuming than I had imagined, with a lot of writing and quizzes. This class taught classical music all the way back to Mozart, musical instruments, and sounds. It was interesting, but I couldn't help thinking about why I was taking this class: for an easier course load. I couldn't complain about the time-consuming schoolwork now; that was life.

The final decision was a tough one: What should I do with the internship? The last free elective was already used for music appreciation. If I were to do the internship, it would have been as a volunteer, and I'd have a long walk a few times a week. My legs were still weak as it was, so that would be grueling. Plus, I still thought that I'd have to devote a lot of my time to the financial management class. I highly valued the experience the internship was going to give me, and I was excited about it. But the question became: Would I rather get experience or would I rather graduate on time? It became clear to me, the internship would only be volunteering and that I needed to concentrate on my studies to make sure I graduated on time.

It turned out to be a wise decision. The next semester was a cold one, and the weather stayed cold through April! It ended up being the norm to see snow on the grass. The fact that the internship location had moved further away meant longer walks in the snow, a few times a week. That would not have been good; I still needed to pass my classes to graduate.

# Chapter Thirteen
# Academic Finish Line

*Good things happen when you*
*least expect them.*
*—Old proverb*

The last semester of my college career had finally arrived. It had been a challenging and interesting road, but now it was time to seal the deal. There were no more options to drop a class and try it next semester; it was important to get through this semester cleanly. This gave me more nervousness, but also more determination. Being determined is important to complete a task, but my nerves had never been this high during my previous semesters.

Regarding the financial management class that I had to retake, I was blessed to find out that my previous financial management teacher, who had been the only teacher for that class the previous semester, had the semester off for a "sabbatical," a period of time where teachers get a break to travel and to research their specialty field. What did I care? The teacher who had given me mental strain was gone! Hallelujah, I caught a big break!

The new teacher I had didn't do quizzes, taught slightly different material and for the second half of the semester, allowed us to use Microsoft Excel on the computer. This was easier and more practical for a person dealing with finance in work. I barely needed assistance from a tutor to pass this class. My new tutor had had the other teacher—the one I wasn't fond of—so it was difficult for him to tutor me, with its being slightly new material and different strategies to complete the questions. I still gave finance a good amount of focus, but not nearly as much as I had to compared to the previous semester.

Academically, it was a great semester. It was filled with lots of group research and presentations. Concentrating more on those two things, rather than on Q&A tests, was a break from the normal college class routine. I did pretty well and dealt with more business classes that prepared me for employment.

## Mix of Timing and Luck

With the groups of people I worked with that semester on different projects, we spent a lot of time together, so I started going out to some bars with them. It was cool; I had some new people to hang out with.

One night I went out with some of my group classmates and my roommate, Tyrone. When I stood with them by the side of the dance floor I noticed something. I could have sworn that I saw Rochelle, the ex-girlfriend from a few years ago, cross by us to walk outside where the smoking section was. She looked really good! Considering this change of events, I did a lot of pondering about the past and about what to do now.

For the next thirty minutes, I was thinking, *Should I talk to her? What do I say? "You look thinner."* No, that's insulting. Finally, I told Tyrone I was going to do it; I was going to talk to her, catch up on things, and compliment her on the fact that she looked good. *That sounds better, doesn't it?*

I open the door to step outside where there was an outside smoking section bar, and I saw the group of girls. I stepped up behind them and said, "Hi, Rochelle." Nobody turned around. Awkward! Maybe they didn't hear me, so I repeated, "Hi, Rochelle."

Finally, the girl turned around and asked, "Are you talking to me?" Then I thought, *How stupid. Rochelle doesn't even smoke!* It was a different girl!

Well, if anything, it was a good and innocent way to start a conversation: Call someone a name and tell her you thought she was someone else. I explained that I thought she was someone I knew. This led me to sit with them. The smoking was bothersome, but it was late and I was pretty loosened up already, so why not?

The girls in this group actually were a couple years older than I was, and I had no idea; two or so years can be easily confused. Oh well, nothing to beat myself up about. The girl I thought was Rochelle, who wasn't, actually had a boyfriend. Any chance with her was gone. But the girl I had called Rochelle told me to talk to her other friend in the group, that she was single. I looked to my right, and she was pretty, so I changed my conversation to talk only to her. We had some stuff in common, enjoyed talking with each other, and found there was a mutual attraction.

Since the conversation was going so well, I put my hand on her waist and went in for a kiss. Her reaction made me surprised and happy at the same time. We did that a few times and continued to get to know each other. Before the night ended, we danced a little bit. Neither of us were great at dancing, so there was nothing for me to be ashamed about. I did notice that we were about the same height; she might have been even a few centimeters taller than me. I thought if I was to continue seeing her, it would give me a good reason to do my chest stretches. A few weeks earlier, my chiropractor had urged me to do chest stretches to make my posture straighter and help get rid of my scoliosis. I thought, *she's pretty and we connected with our conversations. This could be a good thing.* Plus I didn't want to be seen as shorter than her, so figured I'd better start focusing more on my chest stretches.

When I left the bar and said goodbye to the girl at the bar, whose name was Alyssa, I was wondering if I would ever see her again. About twenty minutes after I left, I got a text from her that said, "I already miss you!" Well that answered my question quickly; I'll probably see her soon.

The next night, she drove to my apartment for a few hours. There was one condition; you are not allowed to smoke around me. She understood, and so we enjoyed each other's company again, but this time in a more private setting. Normally I wouldn't wonder about being in a relationship the first night, but I needed to say something because I'm a nice guy. I specifically told her—might I repeat *specifically*—that I wasn't looking for a relationship, with me being in Wilkes-Barre for only three more months. I didn't want to fall for someone and then leave. She agreed and told me about how she was in a relationship with a guy a few years older than her and how that had ended a few months prior. Also, she tried not to date someone younger than her. It surprised her that she was so interested in me, with me being two years younger than her.

For the next few weeks, she came over frequently and we had a good time. But every time I saw her I began to get worried over some things she said. Here are a few questions and remarks she made: Was I pro-choice or pro-life? Would I mind living on the West Coast? Would I be able to deal with her smoking if we lived together? And the list went on. These questions wouldn't have been so alarming if we hadn't already had the conversation about not having a relationship and if it weren't so soon. She really liked me!

Sometimes I spoke about Rochelle to her. For instance, when we walked by the college near King's, the fact that Rochelle used to go to that college, and why I approached her friends at the bar. Alyssa got a little annoyed by it, but, she understood and just reminded me about it, so I would stop. It was weird, because I was more attracted to Alyssa than Rochelle. I didn't think it was that I missed Rochelle; it was more just being reminded of her.

One thing about Alyssa that stood out was that she was incredibly pessimistic about everything. "I have the worst luck with guys; the moon we were born under isn't a good sign, etc." It got tiresome to constantly try to be positive around her negativity.

One time we went out to eat and then she came back to my room for an additional six hours. Tyrone told me, "Dude! You're hurting yourself. You two are in your room for so long and she left at 1:00 a.m. You're leading her on!"

One of my other friends, who was in one of my group projects, said, "I can't wait until it's Facebook official! I'm going to comment 'like' so many times." I told both of them that I already had a talk with her the first night and she agreed this wasn't a permanent relationship. The group project member said, "Okay, but girls like being in a relationship, especially if you see them so frequently."

The next time I saw her things were going okay, but she was acting kind of strange. After we went on a walk, she came into my room and sat on my bed. She asked, "What are we?"

I was surprised she asked that, so I responded, "We're dating, but not in a relationship, as we spoke about that first night. I have no interest in seeing other girls, only you!" Well that wasn't a good enough answer for her! So I had continued to talk to her, puzzled why she was mad. I explained that we had spoken about it in the beginning and wondered why it had to be labeled a relationship. "I told you I didn't want to be in a 'relationship' where I'd open up my heart to you." I'm more cautious on starting a relationship, especially too soon. Plus, my parents live a few hours from Wilkes-Barre and it would be difficult to be in a "relationship." She got over it later that night, but I wouldn't say she was the happiest girl.

After she had left, I texted the friend from my group project, the one who had spoken about a relationship earlier in the day. "Dude, she asked the 'What are we?' question! I hate you for predicting it. Ha-ha. I thought Alyssa and I talked it over in the beginning. I guess she forgot or something." She came over one more time, but Tyrone was complaining that I never hung out with him. I told Alyssa, "I need some bro-time. The next night is ours."

During this "bro-time night," I needed to contemplate what to do with her. I had to call Moe, my friend from home. Remember him from earlier in the book? He was the one who helped me get my first job. Moe was the main person I talked to if I had a question about what to do with girls. He was willing to listen and advise me about girls I was interested in or had dated a few times.

I called Moe and told him the entire story, even the odd questions she asked. He asked, "Could you see her as your girlfriend?"

I responded, "Well I enjoy being around her, we have things in common, I enjoy being intimate, but I don't like that she smokes, the distance, clingy, etc."

Moe said, "I'm not asking you what you like and don't like about her. Can you see her as a girlfriend? Do you see any kind of future with her?"

Finally, I came to my senses, but it was difficult. I didn't want to be in a relationship with her. I told Moe, "No, I'm just going to end it, thanks for the talk."

The next day I still wasn't one hundred percent sure about my decision, but I was leaning towards not seeing her anymore. In one sense, I wanted to see her, but I knew what was right. It was early evening and I was watching a movie with Tyrone. I hadn't texted her all day, because I still wanted to think it over. So she called me and asked if I was all right. I told her that I was, and that I'd call her back in an hour. The hour had passed and I had made my decision to stop seeing her.

I called Alyssa, "Hi. I was thinking it over. Things are just moving way too fast for us." Then I started to list everything that went wrong and started to repeat myself to emphasize it. She cried, "Evan, I get it. You are making it worse! I had feelings in the beginning that it wouldn't work, but I was hopeful that it would. I'll only be okay with it if it's ended mutually." The five-minute conversation ended. I look on Facebook and she had blocked me. I felt that she would appreciate it if I texted her one week later. I put all my thoughts the briefest and kindest way I could. She didn't respond. I wouldn't be surprised if she blocked my number as well. I never talked to her again. I mean, I couldn't if she had blocked me.

## Comical Confrontations

I have a few stories about bouncers and security guards I had confrontations with. I wasn't sure if I was going to write about them, but my mom said they were funny and that I should.

There was this bouncer at one bar who hated me. He noticed that whenever my legs got tired, I'd lean up against the stage to help me stand up. One time when I leaned up against the stage, he and another bouncer approached me and said, "You've had enough to drink. We've been watching you."

Laughing, I replied, "I'm not even drunk. Trust me!" The two bouncers didn't believe me, so each person grabbed the opposite arm and carried me out of the bar.

I looked into the window and saw Tyrone. He came out and yelled, "I told you that they were looking at you and not to lean on the stage. You're not allowed to do that! Your accounting tutor was concerned and asked me to make sure you get home safely."

Another time I went to that same bar with Tyrone. I didn't want to bring my glasses and I was a little tired, since we had walked earlier. All I wanted was to get into the bar/club. In order to get into the place you had to be scanned by a security guard and show the bouncer your ID to prove your age. I wasn't even thinking, so I gave my ID to the security guard instead. Puzzled, he said, "Um, I'm supposed to just scan you for any weapons."

The bouncer next to him told me, "You can't come in. You are drunk."

Tyrone was ready to walk into the place and looked back, noticing that I wasn't allowed in. He just looked at me and said, "Really, Evan? Just follow me next time!"

Later on during my time at college, I mellowed, making sure my legs weren't too fatigued and that I was safe to walk back to my apartment and look sober, which I pretty much was anyway. When I already walked with a little bit of a limp and my legs were already fatigued, it was easy for someone to assume I was drunk.

I had previously worn a white polo shirt to this particular bar/club and it was fine. This time, I wore a different type of white shirt and I wore Mardi Gras beads around my neck. I thought it would look cool; I hadn't worn them in a while, so why not tonight? Tyrone and I went to this bar/club looking to have a good time. Before I could step ten feet from the entrance, the bouncer who hated me stopped me and said, "You're not allowed to wear anything white."

I responded, "I wore white a week or so ago and it wasn't a problem. Is it the beads?"

The bouncer replied, "No. This week we're hearing information from the cops about gang affiliations wearing white."

Tyrone just shook his head and said, "Really, Evan? With all the shirts you have you had to choose white? He doesn't care about the beads around your neck, dude."

One of the last times I was going to go to that same bar/club I went on a long walk with Tyrone. We decided to check the place out; it didn't look too crowded. My legs were tired and I wasn't walking completely straight. My coordination wasn't great and I had difficulty walking in a straight line, even without having had any alcohol.

As we walked to the bouncer who had something against me, he immediately shouted, "You're not allowed in. You aren't walking straight. Too much to drink. I know you."

I thought, *Really? This time I one-hundred-percent did not drink any alcohol.* My legs were tired and I just wanted to see what was up. He was making me angry now. I responded in a loud, firm voice to show that I wasn't stuttering my words, "You idiot—I'm disabled!" The bouncer said, "Oh. I didn't know. Come on in."

## Erase Her

Whenever I engaged with a girl I was interested in, sometimes I would mention Rochelle. Not thinking that I missed her, because I no longer thought she was as attractive as I had in the past; but just that it was the last memory of being in a relationship with a girl in the past year or two.

There was a time in the winter before my final semester that I met a girl from another college and went out to eat with her. She was pretty, but the way her hair, body, and face were shaped was almost one hundred percent like Rochelle. I mentioned Rochelle maybe three times. I felt like I was looking at and talking to Rochelle. After the dinner I was angry at myself. I couldn't understand what was up! It had been a couple years, and I wasn't even interested in her anymore. It must have been a curse or something when opening "Pandora's box" by starting a relationship too soon.

A few weeks after I made my decision to stop seeing Alyssa. I met with two girls and I was attentive to not think of, or mention, Rochelle. From now on, I only wanted to think about whoever I was with or no one at all. When it's the right time for you and your head is focused, seeing other people can be a good way to erase unwanted memories. Take your time moving on, however long it takes. It isn't a race! There is no time limit with moving on and starting to date others; just make sure you're truly ready.

The most important thing was I had never willingly and randomly mentioned Rochelle to a girl or anyone else ever again; so, if there was ever a curse, I must have broken it! The emotions I used to have for Rochelle had been erased from my mind. As to the two girls I just mentioned, I still talk with them occasionally as friends.

Being in a relationship with someone can be complicated. Trauma or no trauma, the ups and downs happen to everyone. With having had a brain injury, maybe her memory was instilled into my brain more. I have no idea. But anyone can have a difficult time letting go of a loved one. Maybe finding a hobby or something to fill your time up will help to distract you. Just let it fade away; try your best to not think of that person or allow your past relationship to creep into your mind again. If you are lucky to have support from peers, embrace it and don't talk about "that person." In fact, erase all contact from that person. That includes their phone number and the texts you shared. Hide or get rid of any material object you have that reminds you of that person. You're just bringing up unwanted memories that can depress you, even though it may not seem good how the relationship ended. But, it may turn out that it was great that it had ended!

# Chapter Fourteen
# Sharing on the Air and Commencing with Life

*Goals are the furnace of achievement.*
*—Brian Tracy*

The day I moved into King's College as a freshman, my dad was proud that I even made it to college after my horrific injury. He had a habit of telling people about my car accident and my remarkable recovery. This annoyed me; I wanted to keep my accident private. I wanted a fresh start, where no one knew of my injury and disability. Plus, I had heard the story *so many* times! And he knew that!

My dad used to play guitar on a semi-professional level when he was younger, and he was pretty good. He was even allowed to play his song, *Fallen Heroes,* in Washington, DC, on the exact date one year after the terrorist attack known as 9/11. He approached the radio station at King's College with one of his CDs, telling me he was going to try to get them to play one of his songs. But he used that as an excuse for going there so he could tell them about my car accident. The radio station was interested in my story and wanted to do a piece about my going to college after the awful accident. Since I wanted a fresh start in college, I declined their offer.

As a junior, I first flirted with the idea about going on their radio station. I found out what the radio station's general email address was, so I sent an email expressing interest. Unfortunately, there was no response. I felt kind of puzzled, but just said, "Oh, well."

Once I reached my senior year, my dad asked me about possibly going on the radio. I told him that I had asked them about it in an email and there was no response. He was confused, wondering why they wouldn't reply; why wouldn't they still be interested in doing a story about me? He had always maintained contact with the manager of King's College radio. He gave me the email address of the station manager, the woman he had spoken to years prior. I decided it was time to see if they were still interested in doing a story about my recovery.

I sent an email to the manager, expressing interest in doing a recovery story. Was she interested this time? Of course, she was. Duh! Sorry—I'm just being sarcastic. She replied to my email immediately. I was excited about that.

The process was that they interviewed me about my car accident, recovery, and going to college. Then they had me interview two friends from home to get their opinion about my car accident and recovery. The two friends I interviewed were Moe and Willis. They did a good job, and I thanked them for letting me interview them. Then I listed two teachers for them to interview.

The student who did the fifty-seven-minute radio story about my recovery, called her radio interview "Reboot: The Evan Higgins Story." "Reboot" was such a good name that I wanted to have it in the title of my book. The reason the radio story was called "Reboot" was because it was something my dad said in his interview about my recovery. As it turned out, the name "Reboot" came full circle, from my dad to the reporter and back to me. It stemmed from when I had no brain flaps to protect my brain for seven weeks and I just lay on the bed doing hardly anything. As my brain swelling started to go down and I started to heal, my brain had to start re-regulating all my bodily functions. Then once I had my skull bone flaps put back in place, that's when my dad coined the phrase, saying that my recovery was like the reboot of a computer. It was then that I was able to begin to function better. Dr. Sugarman did a great job with the operation. I can't thank him enough.

## Oh? I'm Graduating?

My time in college neared the end. It had been full of excitement and stress, but, most importantly, I had learned more about myself. I became more open-minded, with the life experiences of interacting with other people on all levels, and I learned the things that others liked and disliked. In turn, I guess I learned what I liked and disliked also. I'm sure anyone who has attended college can relate to this and wouldn't have it any other way. "College life" helps to prepare you to handle "real life." Yet you can never be fully prepared, because you are always learning new things and those new experiences help to point or guide you in the right direction. In turn, after college you might be more prepared to handle your future endeavors and fulfill what God wants you to do.

I was excited about graduating from college. It was a strange sensation, though—sort of a calm excitement. I wondered, *Why am I not "jumping for joy" excited? I should be. I'm done with undergrad school. I just successfully finished my Bachelor of*

*Science in Business Administration Marketing. This is something to feel proud of; my parents certainly are.* But I couldn't get excited because I was so calm and relieved about passing my classes that semester.

An older person from back home sent me a text to congratulate me. These were some parts of the text that stood out to me: "There is no one on this earth as deserving as you! Stop a moment tomorrow and take it all in... another goal you achieved. I can't wait to see what you do next. Be well." After I read that text I became more excited, but it still hadn't all soaked in yet.

## Today's the Day!

The rewarding day had finally arrived. Graduation! Many colleges call this commencement, the beginning. It was Sunday, May, 18, 2014, the date members of the graduating class of 2014 were given the opportunity to walk down the aisle and receive their diplomas.

My college wanted to make it more special than just walking down the college's gymnasium or outside on a football field to celebrate, I'm sure other college's try be unique, as well. We did it in a hockey arena—how cool is that! I'd never been there, but I had been to arenas to watch professional sports before. The thought of being in an arena with high decks of seats around you and being seen on the jumbo screen accepting your diploma was going to be pretty awesome!

I made sure to get plenty of pictures with my dad! After I walked in my high school graduation in 2009, I didn't want any pictures with him. I was sick of him; I saw him entirely too much in the hospital, and he was extremely protective. He wasn't happy that I didn't want any pictures with him, so a week after my high school graduation I told him, "I'll get a picture with you when I graduate college." When I made that promise, it wasn't even certain that I would be able to get myself to a college level. At that time I was still doing all three therapies as an outpatient at my first therapy place, A.I. duPont Hospital. But my goal was to go to King's College the following year.

There had been some doubt that I would ever go to college. In August 2009 I was permanently home and able to attend a summer school. Summer school was good because I was able to continue to exercise my brain while I was healing. One of my teachers told me I made the right decision, going back to high school and deciding not to get my diploma in June. She didn't necessarily doubt that I was going to go to college, but she talked about my having to be college-ready and that I was far below college level. I told her, "I might have to study more in college, but I'm going next fall."

Back to the person who sent me the text about soaking everything in. After standing in the arena hallway with my classmates for over an hour, waiting for the commencement to finally begin, it started to hit me that I was graduating and I had accomplished the goal I had set five years earlier.

After I saw the introduction of the ceremony and looked up at the jumbo screen where students were starting to receive their diplomas, internally emotions finally started to hit me fully! Unfortunately, because we were a large graduating class, it was over an hour of seeing students walk up on the stage before they got to my section. All the students who were receiving Bachelor degrees in business were in the rear of the seating arrangement and naturally would be receiving their diplomas last. It was difficult to remain excited and joyful for such a long period, so it began to fade away.

But a few minutes before my row stood up I felt that excitement well up again. I walked up the few steps to the stage and received my diploma. Everything was going in slow motion as I accepted the diploma. I gave a long hug to the faculty member who was guiding students where to walk next. This faculty member had seen me recover throughout my college years. She let me know the things I was improving on and guided me in transferring my community college credits that I earned each summer to my King's College credits. I walked back to my seat and waited for the end of the ceremony. It was a great day— a great day to feel accomplishment!

I feel that graduating college is the perfect ending to this memoir. For some time in my life now I thought it would be cool to work with the business and communications sections of a trauma-related healthcare or rehab center. I feel I would be a good asset for them, having recovered from an injury that a lot of families were now facing. The future employment I'll eventually land in is still a mystery, and I'm excited to find out where I will be!

# Chapter Fifteen
## *Final Reflection for You*

*In order to succeed, we must first believe
we can.*
*—Nikos Kazantzakis*

In this last chapter, I want to focus on your getting through tough times in your life. I've heard that some people who have recovered from serious injuries tell people who are going through similar challenges that they should set only small goals. Honestly, I feel that is the wrong approach, because it won't lead you to your true potential. Continuously setting small goals to accomplish can be exhausting, and it doesn't lead you to an end result.

When you're recovering from any type of injury, or even if you're not recovering from anything and just want to accomplish something, set larger goals and set minor goals on the side that lead to the larger ones. Don't be afraid to reach for the stars! If you are in rehab and set a main goal that you want to accomplish, then you will stay motivated to keep going.

For instance, when I was in the hospital my goal was that I wanted to walk. When I first had that passion, I told my physical therapist my goal, though I most certainly wasn't ready to walk quite yet. At that time the opportunity to stand up with assistance was gratifying enough. Standing up was my minor goal. I had to stand before I could walk. Throughout my rehab, if I hadn't had walking in my mind, then I don't believe I would have recovered as fast as I did. In my opinion, yes, the hand you've been dealt can be difficult; but if you believe in yourself and stay highly motivated, nothing can stop you. Only *you* can stop yourself!

With my motivated approach, you've read other examples of my striving to accomplish my goals, whether in walking, swimming, or graduating. But I want to mention something. If there is something you just can't do anymore, it's okay if you can't do it. That sounds hypocritical, doesn't it? All I mean to say is, it's okay to change your goals as new interests and challenges enter your life. Even astronauts and NASA have mid-course corrections. Just make sure you always have a purpose, something you truly want to accomplish.

Was I ever going to be able to swim as fast as I did in the past? That had been my goal early on during my recovery, but I didn't reach that goal. Yes, I was able to race again, but my times weren't as fast as I would have liked. If I devoted my life to swimming, maybe I could have been faster than in the past, but new goals entered my life; I wanted to get stronger. When I started going to college, my swimming activity changed to casually swimming laps in the pool a few times a semester.

When I was a senior, I no longer was as devoted to getting stronger. My college courses had become more time consuming and I wanted to graduate on time. Yes, I still worked out, but I didn't go to the gym as frequently as I had gone in prior years. Old goals keep changing into new goals, so place the previous goals to the side to aim for a bigger or more important current goal.

Do you see my point? You always have to be motivated to accomplish something. If you're not motivated, then nothing will be accomplished. That's when you truly plateau or become stagnant; zero flow of possible improvement! These were the words I hated to hear, and stress that you should hate them, too! If you have no goals to accomplish, then you're pretty much just floating around and doing nothing. I'm the first to admit that there were small times where I felt less motivated or just floated around in life. But every time that happened, I set my mind on something new that I wanted to accomplish. There's always something you can accomplish—don't let a lack of motivation or purpose in life get in your way!

When I was finishing my book, Willis told me, "I believe you got this far because you are stubborn as all hell!" Personally, I think sometimes to get where you want to be you have to be stubborn in wanting to reach your goals. Not letting anything get in your way is an important tactic. Life can be intimidating; just try your hardest to have a purpose in life. And don't let doubters get in the way!

Let's go back to the idea of setting only small goals. To reach your big goals you might get sad at times, but take it step by step. If you continue to set small goals with no big goal or gold star at the finish line, what is it leading you to? Don't you want the satisfaction of reaching each goal you set? It could be anything. Maybe it was the small satisfaction that you were able to accomplish in your one-day diet of not eating sweets. In my case I could not always remember what groceries I needed to get at the store, so I worked on my "grocery store" memory. Whatever your goal is, feel happy you accomplished that!

When your small goal is achieved, now you have to think of another small goal to complete after that. That can become mentally draining and lead you into stagnant points in your life. Ask yourself, does this sound better? "I want to lose ten pounds in two weeks so I'll need to watch what I eat and exercise more." Or "By next week when I go to the grocery store I want to remember my entire grocery list without writing it down on paper." If you think these examples sound better and more gratifying, then setting big goals with small ones on the side is the approach to take. In order to reach those bigger goals, you're going to have to accomplish those small goals first.

I hope my story makes a positive difference for you. Please spread the word about my story to people you think will benefit. You can get through any problem that you face. As my neurosurgeon, Dr. Sugarman, said, "God gave you a second chance in life! He has something very special for you to do! I am going to leave you with the charge to find out what that special thing is. *Go do it.*"

I have heard that when you persevere through a tough situation, you always end up a better person.

# Trauma Notes and Information

Here are a few informative quotes from Brain Injury Alliance, New Jersey, with my comments added.

Traumatic brain injury is an insult to the brain which is caused by an external physical force that may provide a demised or altered state of consciousness, and which results in an impairment of cognitive abilities or physical functioning. It can also result in the disturbance of behavioral or emotional functioning.

Even though I sustained my traumatic brain injury from a car accident, that isn't the only way you can get one. Other examples are from falling, a sports contact injury, shaken baby syndrome, and of course many others. If your brain has any kind of rapid shake, this could result in a trauma to the brain.

Acquired brain injury is an injury to the brain that is not inherited, congenital or degenerative. Acquired brain injuries are caused by some medical conditions, including strokes, encephalitis, aneurysms, anoxia (lack of oxygen during surgery, drug overdose or near drowning), metabolic disorders, meningitis, or brain tumors.

Regarding results of a brain injury, also known as BI:

Whatever the cause, a brain injury can result in an impairment of cognitive abilities and physical functioning.

It can also result in the disturbance of behavioral or emotional functioning. Cognitive consequences may include memory loss, slowed ability to process information, trouble concentrating, organizational problems, poor judgment and difficulty initiating activities. Physical consequences can include seizures, muscle spasticity, fatigue, headaches, and balance problems. Emotional and behavioral consequences can include depression, mood swings, anxiety, impulsivity, and agitation.

Clearly, all brain injuries are different. Different parts of the brain control different parts on our body. That being the case, I feel that for anyone who has had trauma to the brain, the patient's healing time is unknown. People recover at different paces. But always remember, it's important to stay motivated in order to get better.

When I was in the final process of editing my book, I realized something! I didn't really cover or go into great detail about a person's speech after a brain injury. In the beginning of my recovery I tended to speak very quickly. Often, when people listened to me talk, it was difficult to comprehend. Talking slower or faster might be the case for someone with brain trauma.

According to the dictionarist.com, the definition of anomia is "inability to recognize the names of objects and people." Earlier in my recovery, it was difficult to name an object, for example, a pen. But as years passed, I have improved with saying the correct object or name, but not a hundred percent, so it takes me a little extra time to remember a name.

I asked on a few social media pages about misusing words and I got a positive response from people who'd had a TBI. Many of them misspeak words or just can't think of the word to use. Where a brain is damaged can signify how much struggle a person will have with words. But I am certain that people who didn't have brain trauma sometimes make that same mistake, as well. I can assume that everyone misuses words at times; it is just magnified when having brain trauma. When I was younger and didn't have a traumatic brain injury, I know there were times I used the wrong word. If I have any personal advice, I would just keep track of what object and name you struggle with often, so it doesn't remain an issue.

One note that stood out to me from this resource of information was this: "Over 1.7 million Americans sustain a traumatic brain injury every year." Wow, that's a lot, isn't it? More information from the Brain Injury Alliance: "Each year, approximately 80,000–90,000 Americans experience the onset of a long-term disability following a traumatic brain injury, 'TBI.' More than 52,000 people die every year as a result of TBI."

Brain injuries aren't noticed much by society, and that needs to change. A lot of people now are becoming more aware of brain trauma and its seriousness, thanks to the numerous lawsuits from former National Football League players against the League. Their case is that former players were mistreated during games and now they have serious side effects. Sadly enough, that's how society is finding out about brain injuries. It's a big positive that people are becoming more preventative toward brain injuries within sports.

It can happen to anyone and it's incredibly too common! Before my accident, I didn't know anything about brain trauma. But if you are faced with handling a situation along this line, several support groups are available to you, and they can give you more information about this problem. For help on support groups or educational facilities, ask your medical doctor, therapists, school health professional, or someone else you feel is knowledgeable, and search the Internet, too. Other than searching the internet for help, social media is a great way for people to communicate and maybe you could find a social media group or blog that may help.

# Acknowledgments

I want to acknowledge God, friends, family, medical staff, therapists, and teachers. Without you I wouldn't be where I'm at today. The faith, trust, and push you gave me allowed me to reach for the stars.

My dad told me that when I was in the hospital I said, "I want to write a book." That was the first time writing a book came into my mind. But over time the thought of actually writing a book was intimidating and it dimmed out of my awareness. When I was a sophomore in college, though, I had more interest in following through with the book idea. I reached out to my theology teacher, Dr. Thompson, for help and guidance on writing a book. I showed her that I started to write out bullet points of key facts that had happened in my life. She told me I was on the right track and helped to give me a preview about writing a book and figuring out the target audience.

Immediately after college, I began to write my memoir, using bullet points to help me remember what to include. I wrote several drafts before giving it to Carol Sharp, a family friend and an English teacher, the first person to review my book and offer her opinions about it. Then my dad did some revisions with the book and my aunt, Sandy Roth, a professional proofreader, gave me major proofreading and editing assistance. Once I had a satisfied version of the book, Lynette Smith professionally copyedited my book, Howard Harvey created the front and back cover, and my sister Halle Higgins provided the photography on the back cover, and Patsy Bellah formatted the book, and lastly, I would like to give a special thanks to Richard Grungo Jr. for all of his help and guidance throughout my recovery.

To all of you, I extend my heartfelt thanks; without your guidance, my story would never have been told.